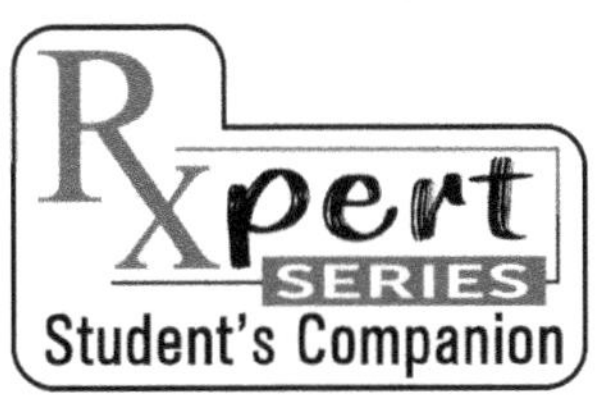

PHYSICAL PHARMACEUTICS – II

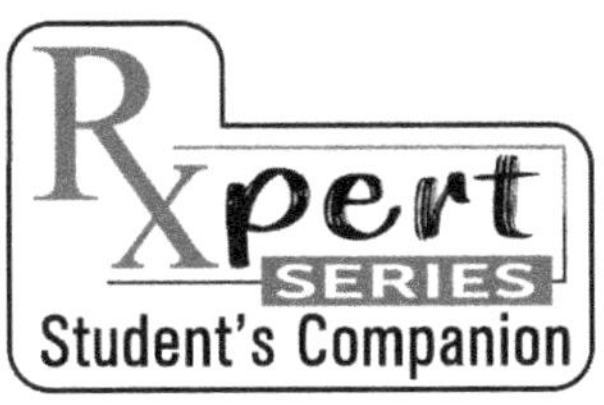

PHYSICAL PHARMACEUTICS – II

Dr. R. Devi Damayanthi, M.Pharm, Ph.D.,
Assistant Professor,
Department of Pharmaceutics,
College of Pharmacy,
Madras Medical College,
Chennai – 600 003, Tamil Nadu, India

Dr. C. Ramasamy, M.Pharm, Ph.D.,
Retd Professor,
Department of Pharmaceutics,
College of Pharmacy,
Madras Medical College,
Chennai – 600 003, Tamil Nadu, India

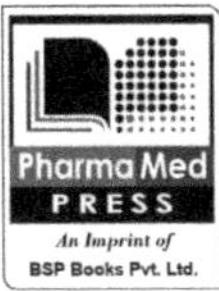

PharmaMed Press
An imprint of BSP Books Pvt. Ltd.
4-4-309/316, Giriraj Lane,
Sultan Bazar, Hyderabad - 500 095.

Physical Pharmaceutics - II

by ***Dr. R. Devi Damayanthi and Dr. C. Ramasamy***

Published by

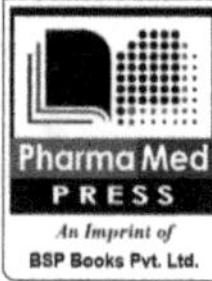

PharmaMed Press

An imprint of BSP Books Pvt. Ltd.

4-4-309/316, Giriraj Lane, Sultan Bazar, Hyderabad - 500 095.

Phone: 040-23445688; Fax: 91+40-23445611

E-mail: info@pharmamedpress.net

www.bspbooks.net/www.pharmamedpress.net

ISBN: 978-93-95039-38-3 (Hardback)

PREFACE

In continuation of Pharmaceutics – I, this book Pharmaceutics – II, has also been written to contain the subject matter in line with the syllabus prescribed by the Pharmacy Council of India. The descriptive manner of the subject topics will help the under graduate students to understand the subject. The inclusion of Addendum with solved problems wherever required, we hope, will help the students to gain some in-depth knowledge and to create interest in the subject and with respect to post graduate students; it may motivate them in doing research work.

Any suggestions for the improvement in the next edition will be wholeheartedly acknowledged with thanks. In this respect, we, in gratitude, expect some positive suggestions.

Dr. R. Devi Damayanthi

Dr. C. Ramasamy

CONTENTS

1. COLLOIDAL DISPERSIONS

Introduction

Particulate systems ordispersions, generally, are of three types – molecular, colloidal, and coarse dispersions. This classification is based on the size of the dispersed particles in the dispersion medium. Blood is a complex dispersed system in which plasma is the dispersion medium. It is composed of almost all the three types of dispersed phases. Nutrients such as peptides, proteins, and glucose form the molecular dispersion. The serum albumin forms the colloidal dispersion and the blood cells such as red blood cells may be considered to form the coarse dispersion.

Colloidal particles in colloidal solution or dispersion have a large specific surface area contributing for their unique properties to be discussed later in this chapter. To understand the increase in surface area, let us consider a cube of 1 cm edge and a volume of $1 cm^3$*. This cube has a total surface area of* $6\ cm^3$*. If this cube is subdivided into smaller cubes with the edge of 100 μm, the total surface will increase by* $600000\ cm^3$*, though the volume remains the same. Thus, specific surface, which is defined as the surface area per unit weight or unit volume, has increased by* 10^5 *times by subdivision of the cube with* $6\ cm^3$*.*

A special significance of colloidal dispersions is that most of of its properties can be used for the determination ofmolecular weight of macromolecules such as proteins and polymers and of theirhomogeneity. For example, insulin is a monodisperse system with a molecular weight of 6000 whereas gelatin is found to be a polydisperse with fractions of molecular weight 10,000 to 100,000g/mole(or daltons). Many of the colloidal solution of polymers are used as viscosity enhancers or viscosity builders in pharmaceutical preparations.

Colloidal dispersions

Colloidal dispersions or *colloids*consist of two distinct phases - a dispersed phase and a dispersion phase or medium. The dispersed phase is also called as internal or discontinuous phase and the dispersion medium, as external or continuous phase or simply medium.

Colloidality is due to a state of subdivision of the dispersed phase. Thus, it is the particle size that distinguishes colloidal dispersions from solutions and coarse dispersions. Dispersed phase in the colloidal state may have the dimensions in the range of 0.001 μ to 0.5 μ.

Solids may be dispersed in colloidal state into paste (zinc oxide in zinc oxide paste and starch in petrolatum,tooth paste containing dicalcium phosphate or calcium carbonate with sodium carboxy methylcellulose) or into liquid (bentonite magma) or into gas (smoke, dust etc.). Liquids may also be dispersed into solid (absorption bases), in aqueous medium (Hydrophilic Petrolatum USP) or in liquid (mineral oil emulsion) or in gas (mist, fog etc.) Gases form colloidal dispersion with solids (solid foam) and with liquids (carbonated beverages).

Molecular dispersion, colloidal dispersion and coarse dispersion from one another may be distinguished as follows:

	Molecular/dispersions (true solution)	**Colloidal dispersions**	**Coarse dispersions**
Size	0.001 micron	> 0.001 micron to 0.5 micron	> 0.5 micron
Visibility	Invisible even in electron microscope	Detected in an ultramicroscope and visible in an electron microscope	Visible to naked eye and in light microscope
Retension	Pass through ultra-filter and ordinary filter paper	Pass through ordinary filter paper but are retained by dialysis or ultrafiltration membrane	Do not pass even through ordinary filter
Diffusion	Undergo rapid diffusion	Diffuse very slowly	Do not diffuse

Note: *1 micron or micrometer*($1\ \mu$) = 10^{-6} *meter* 10^{-3} *mm or* 10^{-4}*cm*

The size of colloidal particles contributes to optical and kinetic properties and the charges present on the particles account for their electrical properties. They usually carry a charge either positive or negative on their surface.

Types of colloids

Colloidal dispersions can be broadly classified into two types - lyophilic and lyophobic. A third type is the association colloid with both the tendencies (i.e., lyophilic and lyophobic). This classification is based on the affinity or interaction between the disperse phase and dispersion medium. (*lyo* means solvent, *philic* means loving, and *phobic* means hating)

1. Lyophilic colloids

When there is considerable interaction (or affinity) between the disperse phase and the dispersion medium, a lyophilic colloid is formed. In this dispersion, the colloidal particles are solvated and they are mostly solids in liquids. Lyophilic colloid may be hydrophilic or lipophilic. If water is the dispersion medium, it is hydrophilic. With lipophilic colloids, non-aqueous vehicle forms the dispersion medium.

Hydrophilic colloids: Hydrophilic colloids may be subdivided as (a) *True solutions*;water-soluble polymers such as acacia and povidone (polyvinyl pyrrolidone) form molecular dispersion in water but the molecules are of colloidal dimensions and hence are classified under colloids. b) *Gelled solutions: These* are solutions of polymers at high concentrations. They are also formed at temperatures at which their solubility in water is low. Solutions of gelatin and starch set to gels on cooling whereas solution of methyl cellulose sets to a gel on heating. If water is the dispersion medium, they are called hydrogels. c) *Particulate dispersions: They* do not form molecular dispersions but they are present as minute particles of colloidal dimensions. Bentonite forms hydrosol with water.

Lipophilic colloids: Lipophilic colloids exhibit affinity for oils and hence are called oleophilic. Oils are non-polar and some examples are mineral oil, vegetable oils such as cotton seed oil and essential oils such as lemon oil. Lipophilic colloids may also be true solutions, gelled solutions or particulate dispersions.

Polystyrene and gum-rubber form colloidal solutions with benzene. Aluminium stearate dissolves or disperses in cotton seed oil. Activated charcoal forms particulate dispersion or sol in all oils.

Lyophilic colloidal dispersions are thermodynamically stable. Lyophilic substances form colloidal dispersions spontaneously with the dispersion medium. They are also reversible i.e. they are again formed after the dispersion medium has been removed i.e. the residue obtained after the removal of dispersion medium forms again a colloidal dispersion on adding to the dispersion medium.

2. Lyophobic colloids

Lyophobic means solvent-hating. In lyophobic dispersions, the colloidal particles exhibit little interaction or affinity with the dispersion medium. Hence in lyophobic collidal dispersions, the particles are not solvated.

Lyophobic colloids may be *hydrophobic and lipophobic*. Hydrophobic dispersion have water as dispersion medium and the particles are not hydrated. Hydrophobic colloids may have lipophilic substances as disperse phase in water. For example, Substance like polystyrene (or gum-rubber), steroids, and magnesium stearate form hydrophobic colloidal dispersions with water. Hydrophobic colloids are formed with substances like gold, silver and sulfur in water.Lipophobic dispersions are water-in-oil emulsions.

3. Association colloids

Association colloids result from the formation of `micelles' (a micelle is formed by a group of surfactant molecules) when a surfactant in sufficient amount is added to the dispersion medium (water). As a surfactant has two distinct portions of opposing affinities (polar and non polar) within its molecule, the molecules tend to associate to form groups called micelles within the medium. The micelles are of colloidal dimensions. Such micelles are formed at and above a concentration called *critical micellar concentration* of the surfactant. Some 50 or more molecules aggregate together to form micelles which are of the order of 50Å (0.005 μ) in diameter. They are thermodynamically stable and also reversible.

Various colloids are differentiated as follows:

	Lyophilic colloid	**Association colloid**	**Lyophobic colloid**
Disperse phase	Consists of large organic molecules of colloidal dimensions or particulate substances.	Consists of aggregate (micelles) of small organic molecules or ions of sub-colloidal sizes. e.g.: surfactants form associated colloids (micelles) in water.	Consists of inorganic particles (i.e., aggregate of atoms; e.g., gold colloid.)
Solvation	Disperse phase particles are solvated with dispersion medium	Hydrophilic portions of the molecule are solvated i.e., hydrated	No solvation (i.e., little interaction between disperse particles and the dispersion medium)
Spontaneity	Spontaneously formed once the disperse phase comes in contact with dispersion medium. They are thermodynamically stable and are also reversible.	Spontaneously formed at and above the critical micellar concentration (CMC). They are thermodynamically stable and are reversible.	Does not form spontaneously but it needs special methods for the formation. Hence they are thermodynamically unstable and are irreversible.
Viscosity due to disperse phase	Viscosity of the dispersion medium is increased. At sufficiently high concentrations they may become a gel. Viscosity is related to the solvation effects and gel formation and to the shape of the disperse phase molecules.	Viscosity increases as micelles increase in number and become asymmetric.	Viscosity is not increased.
Effectof electrolytes	Dispersions are stable generally in the presence of low concentrations of electrolytes. But at high concentrations, the	Electrolytes reduce CMC and at higher concentrations salting out of the disperse phase occurs.	Sensitive even to low concentrations of electrolytes. This is due to neutralisation of

	disperse phase may be salted out (coagulation)		the charge on the colloidal particles. Lyophilic colloids exert a protective effect on lyophobic colloids.

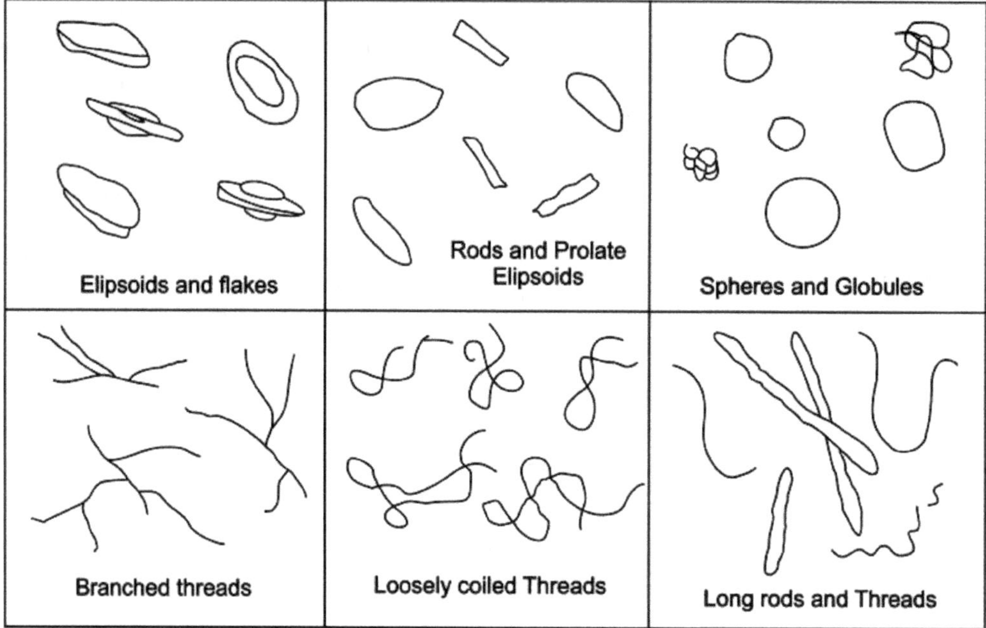

Fig. 1.1. Different shapes of colloidal particles

Properties of Colloids

Properties of colloids may be classified into optical properties, kinetic properties and electric properties.

1. Optical properties

The optical properties may be discussed under Faraday Tyndall effect, electron microscope and light scattering.

(a) The Faraday Tyndall effect

When a narrow strong beam of light is passed through a colloidal dispersion, the path of the light can be observed at right angles under an ultra-microcope. These colloidal particles appear as bright spots against a dark background due to the scattering of light by the colloidal particles on the path of the beam. This optical property is actually due to discrete variations in the refractive index caused by the presence of particles (or by small scale density fluctuations.)

(b) Electron Microscope

The ordinary light microscope cannot reveal the structural details of particles which are separated by smaller distances since the resolving power is about 2000 Å (0.2 μ). The electron microscope has a higher resolving power of about 5Å as it employs electron beam with wavelength of about 0.1Å. The resolving power is directly related to the wavelength of the radiation. The shorter the wavelength, the more efficient is the resolving power.

The electron microscope is used to get pictures of actual particles. It is used to study the size, shape and structure of colloidal particles.

(c) Light Scattering

The scattering of light and the intensity of the scattered light depend upon the following factors.

1. wavelength of the incident beam
2. intensity of incident beam
3. difference in the refractive index between the particles and the medium
4. volume of the particles as well as the number of particles involved in the scattering of light.

The intensity of light scattered may vary at different angles and can be used to obtain some indication as to the shape of the macromolecules (colloidal particles). It may be used to obtain the molecular weight and the equation giving the relationship is given as

$$\frac{Hc}{\tau} = \frac{1}{M} + 2Bc \qquad \text{...(1)}$$

where τ = turbidity measured at 90°to the incident beam.

c = concentration of the solute in grams/liter

M = molecular weight.

B = interaction constant related to the degree of non-ideality of the solution.

H = a constant for a particular system and is given by the equation

$$H = \frac{32\pi^3 n^2 \left(\frac{dn}{dc}\right)^2}{3\lambda^4 N} \qquad ...(2)$$

where n = refractive index

$\frac{dn}{dc}$ = change in refractive index with concentration

N = Avogadro's number

λ = wavelength

A plot of $\frac{Hc}{\tau}$ versus c yields a straight line at low concentration with a slope of 2B. The intercept on the $\frac{Hc}{\tau}$ axis will give the value of $1/M$ and hence the molecular weight.

Light scattering, apart from the molecular weight determination is used for the study of proteins, synthetic polymers, association colloids and lyophobic sols. Light scattering may be used to study the pattern of self-association and it showed that bile salts associate to form dimers, trimers and tetramers. Colloids may exhibit color due to the wavelength of the scattered light. For example, a colloidal dispersion of gold chloride is deep red in color and that of silver iodide is yellow.

2. Kinetic properties

Kinetic properties may be classified as follows:

	Thermally induced	Gravitationally induced	Externally induced
(a)	Brownian movement	Sedimentation	Viscosity
(b)	Diffusion		
(c)	Osmosis		

(a) Brownian motion (or movement)

The macromolecules or the colloidal particles are engaged continuously and randomly in motion within the medium. These molecules or particles are buffeted by the molecules of the dispersion medium. This random movement and bombardment with the molecules of the dispersion medium are increased and become erratic and such a movement of colloidal particles (zig-zag movement) within the medium is termed *Brownian motion*. Brownian motion is decreased by an increase in viscosity of the medium and the motion may also be stopped by increasing this viscosity to a certain level.

(b) Diffusion

Diffusion is a process where the solute molecules move from a region of higher concentration to one of lower concentration until the concentration of the system attains equilibrium and it is due to Brownian motion.

Diffusion is given by Fick's law

$$dq = -DS\frac{dc}{dx}.dt \qquad ...(3)$$

D = diffusion coefficient and is defined as the amount of material diffusing (dq) per unit time across unit area `S' when concentration gradient $\frac{dc}{dx}$ is unity. Diffusion coefficient is a measure of mobility of the dissolved molecules of colloidal dispersion in a liquid medium.

It is possible to compute the molecular weight of approximately spherical particles from the diffusion coefficient by substituting the data obtained from diffusion experiments. The expression to calculate the molecular weight is given as

$$D = \frac{RT}{6\pi r\eta N}\sqrt[3]{\frac{4\pi N}{3M\bar{v}}} \qquad ...(4)$$

Where M = molecular weight

$\bar{v}$ = partial specific volume (volume in cm^3 of 1 g of solute)

η = viscosity of the solvent

R = molar gas constant

T = absolute temperature

r = radius of spherical particle

N = Avogadro's number

Using this method, the molecular weight of egg albumin and haemoglobin have been obtained.

(c) Osmotic pressure

Using osmotic pressure, it is possible to estimate the molecular weight of colloid (colloidal particles) and this is based on Vant Hoff's equation (The osmotic pressure of colloidal solutions is usually very small).

$$\pi = cRT \qquad ...(5)$$

Replacing the c (concentration) with $\frac{c_g}{M}$ the equation is

$$\pi = \frac{c_g}{M}.RT \qquad ...(6)$$

where c_g = gram of solute per liter of solution

M = molecular weight

This equation is valid for very dilute solutions in which the interaction between the solute and the solvent molecules is little and the particles are spherical.

When the solute molecules become solvated (i.e. because of interaction between solute and solvent molecules) there is deviation and the plot of $\frac{\pi}{c_g}$ versus c_g will not be linear and it is necessary to extrapolate the curve to infinite dilution to obtain $\frac{RT}{M}$. The equation is then written as given below when there is interaction between the solvent and the solute molecules.

$$\frac{\pi}{c_g} = \frac{1}{M}RT + Bc_g \qquad ...(7)$$

where B = a constant and is the slope for any particular system and it gives the degree of interaction between the solvent and the solute molecules.

Using this method, the molecular weight of polymers has been obtained.

(d) Sedimentation

Brownian motion keeps the dissolved molecules of colloidal dimensions (macromolecules) or colloidal particles in continuous random motion. Hence it offsets sedimentation due togravity. Therefore, stronger force must be employed to bring about sedimentation of colloidal particles. Even the usual laboratory centrifuges cannot cause sedimentation. This can be undertaken by the use of *ultracentrifuge.* This producessedimentation at a reasonable rate.

In this method, the colloidal dispersion is placed in a glass cell in the ultracentrifuge rotor and arranged in such a way that light passing through the cell may be photographed. The centrifuge is rotated at 50,000 rev/min and higher. The rate of sedimentation is derived from the change in the light absorption or a change in refractive index during centrifugation. The change in refractive index is translated into peaks on a photographic plate. The peaks obtained are termed as *Schlieren patterns* and the peak gives the position of boundary at each time. The boundary (x) refers to the boundary between the solvent and the high molecular weight component (dispersed in the medium) in the centrifuge cell. The boundary and hence the sedimentation is located by a change in refractive index.

Svedberg sedimentation coefficient as it is called is given by

$$S = \frac{\ln\left(\frac{x_2}{x_1}\right)}{\omega^2(t_2 - t_1)} \qquad \text{... (8)}$$

where x_1 and x_2 are measured on the *Schlieren photographs* obtained at times t_1 and t_2. ω is equal to 2π times the speed of the rotor in revolutions per second.

The molecular weight of a polymer is obtained by using the expression.

$$M = \frac{RTS}{D\,(1 - \bar{v}\rho_0)} \qquad \text{... (9)}$$

where R = gas constant

T = absolute temperature

$\bar{v}$ = partial specific volume of the polymer

ρ_0 = density of the solvent

S = *Svedberg sedimentation coefficient* determined at 20°C

D = diffusion coefficient obtained by calculation from diffusion data collected at 20°C

With ultracentrifugation (sedimentation rate method) it is possible not only to determine the molecular weight but also to determine the relative homogeneity of a polymer with respect to molecular weight. If a sample consists of a component of definite molecular weight, the *Schlieren pattern* yields a single sharp peak at any moment during the run. If several peaks appear on the *Schlieren pattern*, it indicates components with different molecular weights. Thus, insulin is found to be a monodisperse (homogeneous) system with a molecular weight of about 6000 and gelatin, a polydisperse system with fractions of molecular weight from 10,000 to 1,00,000.

(e) Viscosity

Viscosity studies provide not only the molecular weight of polymers but also information regarding the shape of the particles in a colloidal dispersion.

Einstein equation provides a quantitative expression for the flow of disperse systems consisting of spherical particles.

$$\eta = \eta_0 (1 + 2.5 \varphi) \qquad \text{... (10)}$$

where η = viscosity of thedispersion

n_0 = viscosity of the dispersion medium

φ = volume fraction ofthe disperse phase (It is the volume of disperse phase divided by the total volume of the system)

The following viscosity coefficients as applied to colloidal dispersions may be defined with respect to Einstein equation.

Relative viscosity η_{rel} is defined as:

$$\eta_{rel} = \frac{\eta}{\eta_0} = 1 + 2.5\,\varphi \qquad \ldots (11)$$

Specific viscosity (viscosity ratio increment) may be defined as the relative increase in viscosity produced by the presence of dispersed phase.

$$\eta_{sp} = \frac{\eta - \eta_0}{\eta_0} = \frac{\eta}{\eta_0} - 1 \qquad \ldots (12)$$

$$\text{hence } \eta_{sp} = 2.5\,\phi$$

In addition, since the volume fraction is directly related to the concentration of the disperse phase, the above equation may be given in the form.

$$\eta_{sp} = Kc \qquad \ldots (13)$$

where K = constant

c = concentration (weight of disperse phase in 100 cm^3 of total dispersion)

The above equation applies to dilute systems only. The equation is usually written as a power series for more concentrated dispersions.

$$\eta_{sp} = \alpha c + \beta c^2 + \ldots$$

Reduced viscosity is obtained by dividing the above equation through `c' and the ratio of specific viscosity to concentration is

$$\frac{\eta_{sp}}{c} = \alpha + \beta c + \cdots \qquad \ldots (14)$$

Intrinsic viscosity $[\eta]$ is the intercept on `y' axis obtained by extrapolating the line obtained by plotting $\frac{\eta_{sp}}{c}$ versus `c' to definite dilution. (Fig. 1.2)

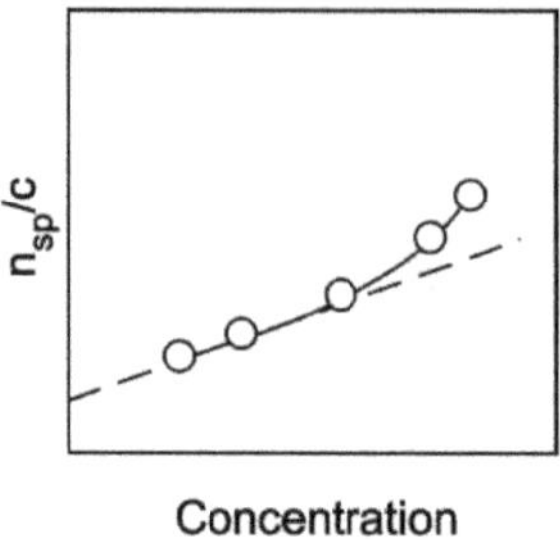

Fig. 1.2

The intrinsic viscosity is used to calculate the approximate molecular weight of a polymer and the equation relating this [η] is given

$$[\eta] = KM^a \quad \dots (15)$$

Where,K and a are constant for a given polymer solvent system and are obtained from other experiments at fixed temperatures. M = molecular weight

This method is used to determine the average molecular weights of starch, dextran and gelatin preparations which are used as plasma extenders. The determination of intrinsic viscosity is used as a test in the BP (British Pharmacopoeia) for the standardization of Dextran injection, a plasma substitute.

The shape of the colloidal particles (disperse phase) influences the viscosity of the dispersion medium. Spherical colloidal particles produce dispersions of relatively low viscosity whereas linear colloidal particles produce dispersions of relatively high viscosity. Viscosity increase is due to salvation effect. When the degree of solvation is more, the dispersion becomes more viscous. Thus, if a linear colloid is placed in a solvent for which it has a low affinity, the linear particles tend to assume a spherical shape and as a result, the viscosity falls. Therefore, the viscosity studies provide a means of detecting changes in the shape of flexible colloidal particles and macromolecules.

3. Electric properties of colloids

The colloidal particles are either negatively charged or positively charged. The particles are negatively charged in kaolin, sulfur, and arsenious sulfide colloidal dispersion while in ferric hydroxide and other metal hydroxide colloidal dispersions, the particles are positively charged. In some other colloidal dispersion such as proteins, the charge of the particles may be positive, negative or neutral depending upon the pH of the medium.

The particles in a colloidal dispersion acquire charges from several sources mainly by ionization or by adsorption

Ionization: A fatty acid soap (sodium stearate), which forms micelles of colloidal size in aqueous solution, ionizes to Na^+ and $C_{17}H_{35}COO^-$ so that the micelle particle carries a negative charge.

Proteins contain both basic and acidic groups in the molecule ($NH_2 - R - COOH$). In alkaline solution, the acidic group - COOH ionizes to $- COO^-$ carrying a negative charge. In acid solution the basic group $- NH_2$ionizes to $- NH_3^+$ so that the particle now carries a positive charge. At an intermediate pH known as iso-electric point, the protein molecule exists as zwitter ion when the net charge is zero provided no other ions are adsorbed. It can be depicted as

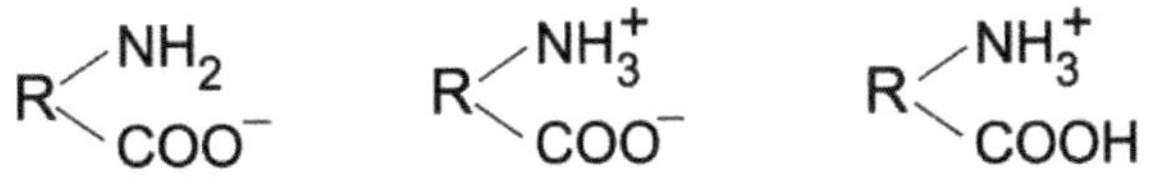

$$R\begin{cases} NH_2 \\ COO^- \end{cases} \qquad R\begin{cases} NH_3^+ \\ COO^- \end{cases} \qquad R\begin{cases} NH_3^+ \\ COOH \end{cases}$$

negative ion — zwitter ion — positive ion

(A protein is least soluble at its isoelectric point and can be readily precipitated.)

*Adsorption:*A non-ionizing colloidal particle may preferentially adsorb ions and thus the particle may acquire a positive or negative charge depending upon which ion (that is anion (–) or cation (+)) is adsorbed. Adsorption of ions, through which particles acquire electric charges usually occur in hydrophobic colloids.

(a) Electric double layer (refer under suspensions also)

The presence of electric charges on the dispersed particles influences the distribution of positive and negative ions in the vicinity of the solution that surround each particle. (Fig. 1.3) Thermal motion also has some influence over the distribution of charges. The resultant effect is that each particle is surrounded by an electric double layer.

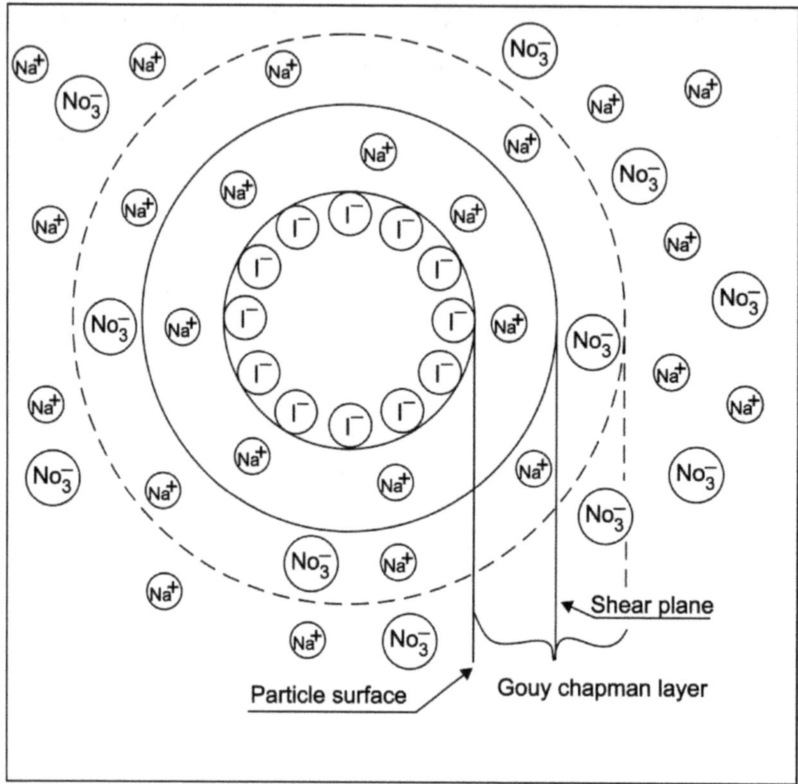

Fig. 1.3

Consider the colloidal dispersion of silver iodide prepared by chemical reaction.

$$AgNO_3 + NaI \dashrightarrow AgI + NaNO_3$$

The colloidal dispersion in water as such will contain Ag^+, I^-, Na^+, NO_3^- and traces of H^+ and OH^- ions.

If the reaction is conducted with an excess of sodium iodide, the surface layer of silver iodide contains more I^- ions than Ag^+ ions and the aqueous solution contains relatively high concentration of Na^+ and NO_3^- ions, a lower concentration of I^- and traces of H^+, OH^- and Ag^+ ions.

As the silver iodide particles contain more of I^- ions on their surface, each of the silver iodide particles is negatively charged and it attracts positive ions from the solution and repels negative ions. As a result, the aqueous solution in the vicinity of the surface (of the AgI particle) contains a much higher concentration of Na^+ ions (called *counter ions or gegenions*) and much lower concentration of NO_3^- ions than in the bulk of the solution. The counter ions Na^+ are pulled closer to its surface and these counter ions tend to stick to the surface as closely as possible as the hydration sphere (the solvated layer on the particle) permits. At the same time, thermal motion (of water molecules) tends to disperse the Na^+ ions throughout the solution. As a consequence, the layer of counter ions surrounding the particle is spread out and however the Na^+ concentration is highest in the immediate vicinity of the negative surface forming a compact layer called Stern layer.The concentration of Na^+ ions decreases with distance from the surface throughout diffuse layer called *Gouy-Chapman* layer. Thus, the negatively charged surface layer is surrounded by a cloud of Na^+ ions (counter ions) required for electro-neutrality. The combination of the two layers of oppositely charged ions constitutes an electric double layer. The thickness of the double layers usually ranges from 10 to 100 Å (0.001 to 0.1 μ)

The presence of electrical double layer around each particle in a colloidal dispersion gives rise to electrokinetic effects. They are electrophoresis, electro-osmosis, sedimentation potential, and streaming potential.

(b) Electrophoresis

When an electric field is applied to a colloidal dispersion, the particles carying the charge (+ or –) move towards the electrode of opposite charge. When the particles move, the counter ions within the hydration shell (i.e., solvation layer) are dragged along with (the surface of the hydration shell is the plane of shear) and the counter-ions in the free or mobile solvent (i.e. medium) move towards the other electrode. This phenomenon is termed *electrophoresis*.

Electrophoretic mobility may be observed using electrophoresis cell. The cell is fitted with two electrodes. After taking a colloidal dispersion in the cell, an electric potential is applied across the electrodes. Under the influence of electric field, the colloidal particles move towards the oppositely charged electrode. The velocity of the particles can be measured by timing their movement. This maybe undertaken by observing through an ultramicroscope (and hence called micro-electrophoresis) which is fitted along with.

The rate of movement of individual colloidal particleis a function of charges on the particle and is directly related to the *zeta potential.* The equation relating zeta potential to the mobility of ion is

$$\zeta = \frac{v}{E} \cdot \frac{4\pi\eta}{\varepsilon} \times (9 \times 10^{4}) \quad \text{... (16)}$$

where ζ = zeta potential in volts

v = velocity of movement of colloidal particles in cm/sec. in an electrphoresis cell of definitelength in cm.

η = viscosity of the medium in poises

ε = dielectric constant of the medium

E = externally applied potential gradient in volts/cm.

$\frac{v}{E}$ = mobility

(9×10^{14}) converts electrostatic units into volts.

When the dispersion medium is water and all the measurement are carried out at 20°C, the equation reduces to approximately

$$\zeta = 150 \frac{v}{E} \quad \text{... (17)}$$

The electrophoretic mobility of colloidal particles can be obtained from the rate of movement of the boundary of a sol using a simple `U' tube apparatus. This method is called *moving boundary electrophoresis* and is used when the particles cannot be observed individually with an ultramicroscope. In moving boundary electrophoresis, a sharp boundary is formed between the sol and the pure dispersion medium and its movement in an electric field is observed visually if the disperse phase is colored. If the disperse phase is colorless, the boundary is observed by a change in refractive index along the column using special optical equipment (*Schlieren method*).

This method permits the identification of different colloidal components in a mixture, to study the electrophoretic mobility of the components in the mixture (e.g. proteins) and to estimate the relative amounts present.

(c) Electro-Osmosis

If the charged colloidal particles are rendered immobile, the counter-ions in the free water (dispersion medium) move towards the electrode of opposite charge dragging the water along with. This flow of liquid medium under the influence of electric field is called electro-osmosis and is considered to be opposite in principle to that of electrophoresis. The pressure produced by the process of electro-osmosis is called *electro-osmotic pressure.*

The atmosphere of counter-ions around the particles (apart from the counterions present within the hydration shell of the charged colloidal particles) confers a charge on the dispersion medium. This causes the liquid medium to move towards the opposite electrode under the influence of electric field. This phenomenon can be observed if the tube containing the colloidal dispersion is plugged in the middle with a porous material and across which a potential is applied. This method (electro-osmosis) also provides for obtaining zeta potential.

(d) Streaming potential

It is the converse of electro-osmosis. In this a potential difference is created, if the liquid is forced to flow past a plug or bed of charged particles by applying hydrostatic pressure. The potential difference is created because of the displacement of counterions in the free water. This method too can be used to determine the zeta potential.

(e) Sedimentation potential

This is the reverse of electrophoresis. When the colloidal particles are caused to undergo sedimentation, a potential difference is created.

(f) Donnan Membrane Effect

The presence of charged macromolecules (colloid) on one side of a semipermeable membrane (impermeable to macromolecules) will affect the diffusion of smallions (may be drug ions) through the semipermeable membrane. This effect is due to the electrical gradient across the membrane and as a consequence, the charged drug ions of the same charge as that of macromolecules are driven to the opposite side of the membrane altering the concentration of the drug ions. This is termed *Donnan membrane equilibrium* or simply *Donnan effect* and may be demonstrated as follows.

Suppose a colloidal solution, the colloidal particles of which carrying negative charges together with its counterions say R^-NA^+ contained in a semipermeable membrane sac is placed in a solution of a drug (such as sodium salicylate) which has ionized into positive and negative ions say Na^+andD^-. Considering the volumes of solutions on the two sides of the membrane (i.e. inside and outside) are equal, the system at equilibrium is represented as follows

Outside	**Inside**	
(o)	**(i)**	
Na^+	R^-	$\begin{bmatrix} Na^+ \\ D^- \end{bmatrix}$ Permeable ions
D^-	Na^+	R^-- Non-Permeable ion
	D^-	

In accordance with the principle of escaping tendencies, the concentration of the drug (Na^+D^-) must balance on both sides of the membrane. i.e.

$$[Na^+]_o\,[D^-]_o = [Na^+]_i\,[D^-]_i \qquad \text{... (18)}$$

where subscripts o and i indicate outside and inside respectively.

Applying electroneutrality on both sides,the concentration of positively charged ions must balance the concentration of negatively charged ions

i.e., outside: $[Na^+]_o = [D^-]_o$

and inside: $[Na^+]_i = [R^-]_i + [D^-]_i$

Substituting these in the equation (18) we obtain

$$[D^-]_o\,[D^-]_o = ([R^-]_i + [D^-]_i)\,[D^-]_i$$

$$[D^-]_o^2 = [R^-]_i\,[D^-]_i + [D^-]_i\,[D^-]_i$$

$$[D^-]_o^2 = [D^-]_i^2 + [R^-]_i\,[D^-]_i$$

$$= [D^-]_i^2\left(1 + \frac{[R^-]_i}{[D^-]_i}\right)$$

$$\frac{[D^-]_o^2}{[D^-]_i^2} = 1 + \frac{[R^-]_i}{[D^-]_i} \qquad \text{... (19)}$$

or $$\frac{[D^-]_o}{[D^-]_i} = \sqrt{1 + \frac{[R^-]_i}{[D^-]_i}}$$

From the above equation which represents the ratio of concentrations of diffusible drug anion outside and inside the membrane at equilibrium, it may be understood that a charged polyelectrolyte (i.e., macromolecules of colloidal dimensions) inside a semipermeable membrane sac would affect the equilibrium concentration ratio of a diffusible anion. That is it tends to drive the ion (drug ion) of like charge on its side to the opposite side through the semipermeable membrane. It is simple mathematics that when $\frac{[R^-]_i}{[D^-]_i}$ is equal to 15, the ratio of $\frac{[D^-]_o}{[D^-]_i}$ is equal to 4 and when $\frac{[R^-]_i}{[D^-]_i}$ is equal to 120, the ratio $\frac{[D^-]_o}{[D^-]_i}$ will be equal to 11. Thus, the addition of an anionic polyelectrolyte such as sodium carboxy methyl cellulose to a diffusible drug anion such as potassium benzyl penicillin and sodium salicylate enhances the diffusion of drug and thereby increases the absorption. The presence of charged electrolyte not only influences the distribution of drug ion according to *Donnan equilibrium* but will bring about an increase in the rate of transfer of the drug across the membrane.

It was also found that ion exchange resins, sulfate and phosphate ions which do not diffuse through intestinal wall, will drive anionic drug from the intestinal tract into the blood stream.

[Note: Charges on the membrane also influence the permeability of anions and cations. For example, a collodion membrane which possesses fixed anions and mobile cations will be selectively permeable to cations and the anions being repelled by negatively charged membrane.

Conversely, a membrane with fixed cations and mobile anions will be selectively permeable to anions]

Preparation of Colloids

1. Lyophilic colloids

Owing to the affinity of lyophilic colloids for the dispersion medium, these colloidal sols are formed with relative ease. As there is considerable interaction between the disperse phase and the liquid dispersion medium, (i.e., there is extensive solvation) lyophilic dispersions are formed spontaneously when the material is placed in contact with the liquid. They are thermodynamically stable and reversible.

Acacia and povidone will readily disperse if added to water forming a colloidal solution. Gelatin and starch form colloidal sols spontaneously (especially in hot water) with water.

2. Lyophobic colloids

Most of the lyophobic dispersions are hydrophobic dispersions. They include aqueous dispersions of insoluble organic and inorganic compounds which have a low degree of hydration (i.e., less interaction).

Because, hydrophobic dispersions are intrinsically unstable and there is little interaction between the disperse phase and the dispersion medium (water), preparation of hydrophobic colloids needs special methods. They can be prepared by *dispersion or condensation*. Dispersion methods involve breaking up of disperse phase to small particles of colloidal dimensions through milling and grinding (particle size reduction or comminution) or peptization. Condensation methods involve the aggregation of small molecules or ions to produce particles of colloidal dimensions.

Comminution

Comminution can be carried out by two methods

(a) *Dispersion methods*: Colloid mills, ball mills and micronizers can be used to reduce the size of particles to colloidal range. In a colloid mill, the coarse material is sheared in a narrow gap between a static cone and a rapidly rotating cone to colloidal sizes.

In electrical dispersion method (*Bredig's arc method*) the dispersions of metals are prepared by producing an electric arc by keeping close together two electrodes made of the metal immersed in water containing traces of KOH as stabilizer in a container cooled by ice externally. The intense heat vaporizes some of the metal and the vapor condenses into colloidal particles in water. Eg. silver, gold, platinum hydrosols.

Colloidal dispersions of many materials such as sulfur and graphite can be obtained by means of ultrasonic waves. Emulsification by ultrasound waves is the method of choice for the preparation of soyabean oil emulsion in water for intravenous injection.

(b) Peptizationis a process of dispersion of a precipitated material (flocculated or aggregated) into smaller aggregates of colloidal dimension.

It can be effected by the addition of deflocculating or peptizing agents. Peptizing agents may be surfactants, water soluble polymers, or ions which are adsorbed at the particle surface and they do not allow aggregation and keep the particles in the colloidal dimensions. Peptization occurs in the presence of an electrolyte carrying the same ion or charge as that of the precipitated particles. It is usually undertaken with freshly precipitated particles. For example, when a small volume of very dilute solution of hydrochloric acid is added to a fresh precipitate of silver chloride, it leads to the formation of colloidal solution of silver chloride.

Peptization can also be brought about by the removal of flocculating agents (electrolytes) and their removal results in the disintegration of floccules into small particles of colloidal dimensions. Even washing the gelatinous precipitate of aluminium hydroxide with water bring about peptization. Ferric hydroxide yields a sol when ferric chloride (Fe^{3+} being common ion) is added to it.

Condensation methods

A change in solvent may bring about the formation of colloidal particles by condensation. If an alcoholic solution of resin is poured slowly into water, a colloidal dispersion of resin in water is obtained. In the same manner, when an alcoholic solution of sulfur is mixed with water a bluish white colloidal dispersion of sulphur is produced. This is usually undertaken in the presence of a stabilizing agent to prevent precipitation.

Colloidal dispersion may be obtained by chemical reaction also. Colloidal sulphur may be obtained by bubbling hydrogen sulfide gas into an aqueous Sulphur dioxide solution

$$2H_2S + SO_2 \longrightarrow 3S + 2H_2O$$

Colloidal dispersions of aluminium hydroxide may be prepared by hydrolyzingaluminium chloride

$$AlCl_3 + 3H_2O \longrightarrow Al(OH)_3 + 3HCl$$

By double decomposition of sodium chloride with silver nitrate, a colloidal dispersion of silver chloride may be obtained.

$$NaCl + AgNO_3 \longrightarrow AgCl + NaNO_3$$

A colloidal dispersion of ice in ether or chloroform can be obtained by freezing saturated solution of organic solvent in water.

Purification of colloidal dispersion

Most of the hydrosols contain low molecular weight water soluble impurities. Presence of electrolytes as impurities in hydrophobic dispersion has to be avoided as it may coagulate such dispersions. These dissolved impurities are removed by dialysis, electrodialysis and ultrafiltration. However, traces of electrolytes are needed to stabilize the colloidal system.

(a) Dialysis

It is a process based on unequal rates of passage of solutes and solvent through microsporus membrane.

Dialysis can be simply carried out by placing the colloidal sol in a *cellophane sac* and immersing this sac into a large vessel of water. Low molecular weight solute molecules diffuse out into water while the colloidal particles remain inside the sac entrapped. Dialysis rate may be increased by increasing the area through which diffusion occurs, by stirring, and by maintaining a high concentration gradient across the membrane. To maintain a high concentration gradient, the water is replaced continuously or changed repeatedly. Diffusion is continued until the colloidal sol is substantially free form the low molecular weight solute molecules.

Ordinary dialysis is relatively slow and if electrolytes of low molecular weight are the impurities to be removed, the process of dialysis can be speeded up by applying an electric potential. This technique is called electrodialysis.

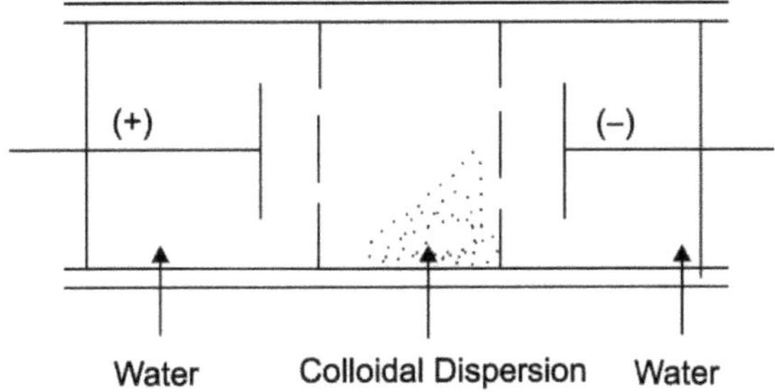

Fig. 1.4 Electro-dialysis cell

An electrodialysis cell consists of three compartments two outer and one center compartment. (Fig. 1.4) The center compartment is separated from the two other compartments on either side by two dialysis membranes supported by screens. The two outer copartments contain water and also the electrodes and the center compartment the colloidal sol. When an electric potential is applied, the anions move from the sol into the anode compartment while the cations move from the sol into the cathode compartment. The colloidal particles in the center compartment move towards one of the membranes according to the charge they carry. Non electrolyte solute molecules (impurities) diffuse into both the outer compartments. As the density increases due to the accumulation of colloidal particles, they settle to the bottom of the center compartment as shown in Fig.1.4. The supernatant liquid can be changed by decantation and thus the purified colloidal sol is prepared by electrodialysis and decantation. This process is called *electro-decantation.*

(b) Ultrafiltration

Keeping the colloidal sol in a compartment that is closed by a dialysis membrane of pore size 0.003 μ and applying pressure, the liquid and the low molecular weight solute molecules are forced through the membrane. The colloidal particles are retained within the compartment. This separation process is called *ultrafiltration*. Ultrafiltration differs from dialysis only in that the passage of the small molecules of low molecular weight through the membrane is enhanced by applying usually high positive pressures. As the process uses high pressure, the membrane is usually supported by a fine wire screen.

In order to avoid the increase in the concentration of colloidal particles and to remove the dissolved impurities completely, the water is replaced continuously or repeatedly by equal amounts of de-ionized water. To maintain uniform concentration throughout the colloidal sol, the sol is stirred.

Ultrafiltration has been used to separate and purify colloidal sols. An ultrafilter may be an ordinary filter paper impregnated with collodion (Cellulose tetranitrate dissolved in a mixture of ether and alcohol in the ratio of 3:1) or cellophane (a regenerated cellulose in swollen gel sheet) or cellulose acetate.

Stability of Colloids

The stability of a colloidal dispersion depends on two factors

1. presence of charge (+ or -) on the dispersed colloidal particles
2. Solvent sheath surrounding each dispersed particle

When the colloidal particles collide as a result of *Brownian movement*, the above two factors will prevent mutual adherence. It may be said that the stability of lyophobic colloid is largely due to the electric charges on the surface of the dispersed particles and for lyophilic sols it is the solvent sheath that is significant in stabilizing the system.

In a lyophobic sol as already mentioned, the particles are stabilised by the presence of electric charges on their surfaces. The like charges present on their surfaces prevent the coagulation of the particles. Coagulation is a process where the colloidal particles aggregate together resulting in the precipitation of the dispersed particles and ultimately the colloid dispersion breaks up i.e., becomes unstable. Coagulation (or aggregation of colloidal particles) may be brought about by the addition of electrolytes which reduce the zeta potential (the sign and magnitude of charge on the particle). The coagulating power of electrolytes depends on the valency of the active ion (ion causing coagulation). The higher the valency of the ion, the greater is the precipitating power. This is known as the *Schulze-Hardy* rule.

The stability of lyophobic colloids is described by DLVO theory *(Derjaguin, Landau, Verwey and Overbeek)*. The forces operating on colloidal particles in a dispersion are the repulsive and attractive forces. The repulsive forces are due to overlapping of electrical double layer and the attractive forces are due to London type *van der Waals* forces. The potential energy of repulsion (V_r) is shown in Fig. 1.5 and also the potential energy of attraction V_a. V_0 indicates the composite potential energy, (i.e. interaction curve).

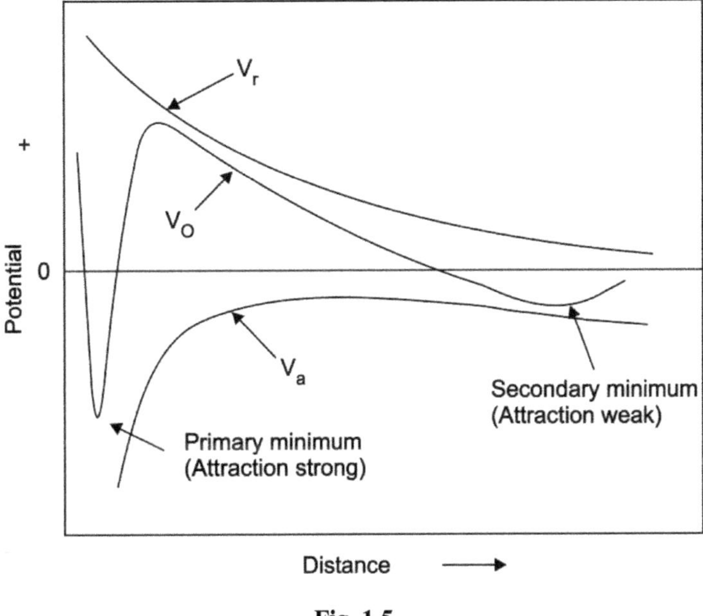

Fig. 1.5

As two particles approach each other in the medium a weak attractive force exists beyond the range of electrical double layer repulsive forces. This attractive region is called the *secondary minimum*. It is responsible for flocculation. This is significant in the controlled flocculation of suspended particles in a coarse dispersion (a suspension). If the thermal energy is equal or greater than the repulsive barrier (V_r) the particles come closer and encounter strong attraction in the *primary minimum* shown in the figure. When the particles get into the primary minimum, they coagulate.

At low electrolyte concentration, the repulsive forces predominate so that the particles experience only a repulsive force upon approach. The particles remain individually and the system is called dispersed or peptized. At a high concentration of electrolyte, the electrical double layer forces are greatly diminished. As a result, *van der Waals* forces of attraction predominate and the particles encounter net attractive forces ending in coagulation.

Lyophilic and association colloids are thermodynamically stable and they exist in true solution. Hence, they do not coagulate on the addition of moderate amounts of electrolytes. However they coagulate if sufficient amount of electrolyte is added. This is termed `salting out'. The coagulating power in lyophilic colloids may be given by *Hofmeister or lyotropic series.* Anions of Hofmeister series in decreasing order of precipitating power are citrate, tartrate, sulfate, acetate, chloride, nitrate, bromide and iodide. The precipitating power is due to their ability to dislodge solvent sheath from the colloidal particles.

Even the addition of solvents such as alcohol and acetone which are having greater affinity to water causes coagulation of colloidal particles. Addition of such solvents lowers the dielectric constant of the medium which is unfavorable for the colloidal particles.

Coacervation

When oppositely charged hydrophilic colloids are mixed, the colloidal particles may get separated forming colloid-rich layer. Such a formation of colloid-rich layer is termed as coacervation. The process of formation of coacervates is called coacervation. For example, Gelatin and acacia in water form hydrophilic colloids. Gelatin is (below pH 4.7) is positively charged while acacia is negatively charged. If these two oppositely charged colloidal solutions are mixed at a definite proportion, coacervates are formed. Coacervation may also be brought about by the addition of alcohol, sodium sulfate or starch.

When a polar solvent such as alcohol or acetone is added to a hydrophilic colloid, (i.e., a colloidal dispersion in more polar solvent such as water), it will decrease the solubility of colloidal particle in water. To this if a small amount of an electrolyte is added, it may bring about the coagulation or flocculation of the colloidal particles. It may be regarded that flocculation is a transformation of a sol hydrophilic nature to one of more hydrophobic nature.

This coacervation process forms the basis for microencapsulation of drug products. Thus, sulfamethoxazole drug particles can be encapsulated with gelatin-acacia coacervates. An aqueous mixture of sulfathiazole and povidone also results in coacervation by the addition of resorcinol, a coacervating agent for povidone.

Using microencapsulation process to different thicknesses, sustained release dosage forms, which have wide commercial applications, are manufactured.

Sensitization and Protection

When a small amount of hydrophilic or hydrophobic colloid is added to a hydrophobic colloid of opposite charge, the hydrophobic colloid becomes sensitive.

Sensitization is attributed to a reduction in zeta potential below the critical value (the value below which coagulation occurs). It is also reasoned that it is due to a reduction in the thickness of the ionic layer surrounding the colloidal particles.

However, addition of large amounts of hydrophilic colloid tends to stabilize the system because of adsorption of hydrophilic colloid particles forming a protective cover on the hydrophobic colloid particles. This phenomenon is called *protection*. The hydrophilic sol used for the purpose of protecting the hydrophobic colloid is known as protective colloid. This protective power of hydrophilic colloid may be given in terms of "*gold number*".

The *gold number* is the weight in milligrams of the protective colloid (on dry basis) needed to prevent a color change from red to violet in 10 ml of gold sol on the addition of 1 ml of 10% solution of sodium chloride. Gold numbers of some protective colloids are given below.

Protective colloid	Gold number (mg)
Gelatine	0.006 - 0.01
Albumin	0.1
Acacia	0.1 - 0.2
Tragacanth	2

2. RHEOLOGY

Introduction

Rheology is the science of flow of materials under stress. Flow property of materials is mainly of two types – Newtonian and non-Newtonian. In the case of Newtonian flow, the viscosity of materials remains the same whatever be the stress applied. The Newtonian systems may be of different viscosities from low viscosity (such as water) to high viscosity (such as honey). The difference in viscosities is due to differences in the resistance offered to the flow by the respective liquid.

The Newtonian systems are again put into different types namely dilatant, plastic, and pseudoplastic systems. Dilatant systems or materials flow immediately once the stress is applied but as the stress is increased, the apparent viscosity of the system increases. At very high stresses the viscosity increases to a greater extent and at high stresses the flow may even stop damaging the stressing system.

The pseudoplastic system also flows immediately once the stress is applied but, in this case, the viscosity decreases on increasing the stress. The plastic system differs from pseudoplastic system by not flowing until a certain minimum stress is not exceeded i.e., the system does not flow at initial mild stresses. The flow occurs only after a minimum stress is exceeded and on further increasing the stress, the viscosity decreases as in the case of pseudoplastic systems. The minimum stress above which the flow starts is termed as yield value. Once the yield value is exceeded, the system starts to flow and on increasing the stress further, there is decrease in viscosity as in the case of pseudoplastic systems. Within the yield value, the plastic system behaves like elastic system. The yield value in plastic systems can be considered as elastic limit. Once this limit is exceeded, the flow starts and on increasing the stress, the viscosity decreases,

Even solids (powders) flow under stress and in this case, there is elastic and plastic flow. Elastic flow refers to the point within which, the solid will regain its original shape on removal of the stress applied. Once the stress is exceeded greater than the elastic limit, there occurs what is called plastic flow which is irreversible and it ultimately leads to complete deformation. These behaviors assume importance when pharmaceutical powders are subjected to stress to form tablets and the properties of tablets depend on the elastic and plastic deformation.

Rheology

The term rheology was derived from two Greek words namely *rheo* (to flow) and *logos* (science). Rheology is the science that deals with the deformation of matter under the influence of stresses. The stresses may be

(a) *Tensile stress:* a stress applied perpendicularly to the surface of a body

(b) *Shearing stress:* a stress applied tangentially to the surface of a body.

(c) Stress applied at any other angle to the surface of a body can be merely called as *stress*.

The deformation is of two types.

Elastic deformation	Plastic deformation
It is spontaneous and reversible. The work spent for the deformation is recoverable when the body returns to the original position.	It is permanent and irreversible. The work spent for the deformation is dissipated as heat.

The flow properties or viscous behavior of various pharmaceutical products ranging from simple liquids to semisolids such as ointments, gels, creams and pastes are very important for pharmacists in the following areas as detailed below.

1. For fluids

- Mixing of liquids
- Particle size reduction of disperse system with shear.
- Passage through orifices, including pouring, packaging in bottles, and passage through hypodermic needles.

- Fluid transfer, including pumping and flow through pipes
- Physical stability of disperse systems.

2. For semisolids

- Acceptable consistency and smoothness
- Spreading and adherence on to the skin
- Removal from jars or extrusion from tubes
- Capacity of solids to mix with miscible liquids.
- Release of the drug from the base
- Mixing and packing into containers.
- Physical stability and patient acceptability
- Biological availability from skin and gastro-intestinal tract

3. For solids

- Flow of powders from hopper and into die cavities in tableting and flow of powder into capsules during encapsulation.
- Packageability of powdered or granular solids.

4. Processing

- Production capacity of equipment
- Processing efficiency
- Correct choice of production equipment.

Viscosity

Viscosity is qualitatively defined as the resistance of a liquid to flow due to internal friction between different layers of liquid when it flows.

It may be treated mathematically as follows.

When the liquid flows (e.g., liquid passing through a pipe) due to a shearing stress, a plastic deformation occurs. Due to this, there is a change of velocity between different layers of the liquid. That is, the velocity changes from zero (liquid at the periphery of the pipe) where the distance $x = 0$ from the base to a maximum value u at the topmost layer. (In the case of liquid flowing through a pipe, the velocity will be maximum at the center of the pipe Fig. 2.2).

Let us consider the liquid is made up of infinitely thin parallel layers (laminae) each of area A on a horizontal base as shown in (Fig. 2.1). u

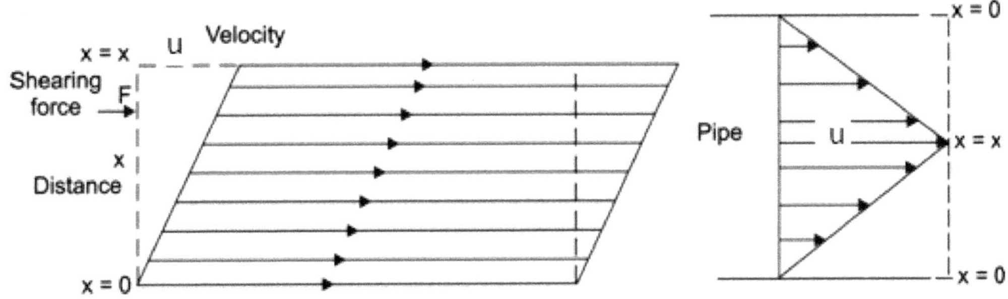

Fig. 2.1 **Fig. 2.2**

Representation of movement of a liquid in a planar lamina and through a pipe

The infinitesimal difference of velocity du between two layers of liquid separated by an infinitesimal distance dx is the velocity gradient and the change in velocity with distance is the rate of shear and is given by $\frac{du}{dx}$. The force per unit area required to produce a certain rate of shear is called the shearing stress, S, i.e., $S = \frac{F}{A}$.

Shearing stress and shear rate are related by $S \propto \frac{du}{dx}$.

Introducing proportionality constant

$$S = \eta \frac{du}{dx} \qquad \text{... (1)}$$

or

$$\eta = \frac{\text{shearing stress}}{\text{rate of shear}} = \frac{S}{du/dx}$$

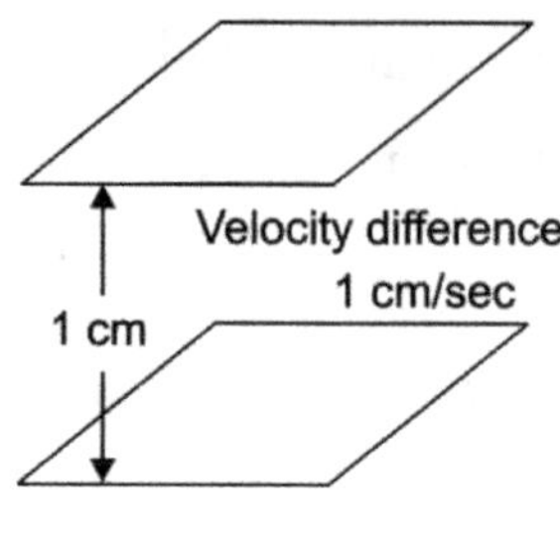

Fig. 2.3

It may also be defined as the force (in dyne/square centimeter) required to maintain a velocity difference of 1cm/sec between two parallel layers of liquid of each one square centimeter separated by a distance of 1 centimeter (Fig. 2.3). If the force required is 1 dyne/square centimeter, the coefficient of viscosity or simply viscosity (η) is said to be one poise (P)

The unit may be obtained by dimensional analysis

$$1 \text{ poise} = 0.1 \text{ Nsm}^{-2}$$

$$\eta = \frac{F}{A} \cdot \frac{dx}{du} = \frac{\text{dyne } \times \text{cm}}{\text{cm}^2 \times \text{cm/sec}} = \frac{\text{dyne sec}}{\text{cm}^2}$$

(i.e. 0.1. Newton second per square meter)

Newton second is the SI unit for poise.

Dyne.sec/cm^2 can also be given as g/cm.sec, since, $\frac{dyn.sec}{cm^2} = \frac{g \times \frac{cm}{sec^2} \times sec}{cm^2} = \frac{g}{cm.sec}$

Liquids showing high coefficient of viscosity is said to be viscous and the liquid showing less coefficient of viscosity is said to be less viscous or mobile. For mobile liquids, the convenient unit is *centipoise* which is one hundredth of 1 *poise*. The reciprocal of viscosity is called fluidity (ϕ). (The unit is Poise^{-1})

$$\phi = \frac{1}{\eta} \quad \text{... (2)}$$

Kinematic viscosity

Kinematic viscosity is the absolute viscosity (η) divided by the density of the liquid. The units are *stoke* and *centistoke*.

Viscosity of liquids

Poisuille was the first scientist who designed an equipment to find out viscosity of liquids. The equipment consists of a tall cylinder attached with a capillary flow tube at its lowest side at right angle to it (Fig. 2.4).

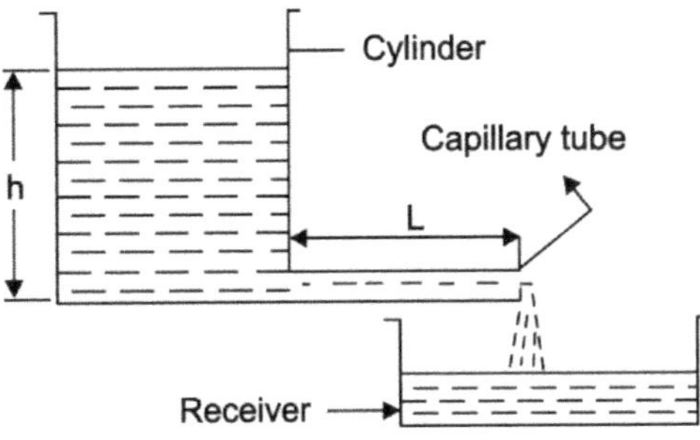

Fig. 2.4

The liquid is filled up to the height 'h' in the cylinder and a specified volume of liquid is collected into a reservoir through the capillary tube of length l and radius 'r'. Then, the volume of liquid collected is given by

$$V = \frac{\pi p r^4 t}{8\eta l} \quad \text{... (3)}$$

where V = volume of liquid collected

p = pressure head due to the liquid and is equal to '*hdg*',

i.e. height × density × acceleration due to gravity.

r = radius of the capillary tube.

t = time upto which the liquid was collected.

η = coefficient of viscosity of the liquid.

l = length of the capillary tube.

Rearranging the formula for (η) (viscosity),

$$\eta = \frac{\pi}{8}\frac{pr^4 t}{Vl} \quad \text{... (4)}$$

in which all the parameters are measurable and η can be calculated easily.

Effect of temperature on viscosity

It is fact that as the temperature of a system is increased. viscosity decreases. Approximately for one degree centigrade rise, the viscosity falls by 1 to 10%. It is mathematically given as

$$\eta = Ae^{E_a/RT} \qquad ...(5)$$

Or

$$\ln \eta = \frac{E_a}{RT} + \ln A \qquad ...(6)$$

where A = a constant

R = gas constant

T = thermodynamic temperature

E_a = energy of activation to move one molecule past another

However, there are some exceptions. For example, viscosity of methyl cellulose solution *increases* as the temperature *increases.*

Hence the viscosity is affected by temperature, it is necessary to report the viscosity of a system at a given temperature and in the determination of viscosity of substances, the temperature should be maintained constant throughout the experiment.

Types of Rheological Systems

It is broadly classified into two types

I. Newtonian systems

II. Non-Newtonian systems.

1. Newtonian systems

Rheological properties of a system are usually expressed in the form of a graph wherein shearing stress (on the x axis) is plotted against rate of shear (on the y axis) and this is called a *rheogram.*

If a system shows same values of 'η' (i.e., coefficient of viscosity) at different shearing rates at a given temperature, it is said to be a Newtonian system.

S.No.	Shearing stress	Shear rate	$\eta = \frac{Shearing\ stress}{shear\ rate}$
1	x_1	y_1	$\frac{x_1}{y_1} = n$
2	x_2	y_2	$\frac{x_2}{y_2} = n$
3	x_3	y_3	$\frac{x_3}{y_3} = n$
.	.	.	.
.	.	.	.
.	.	.	.
n	x_n	y_n	$\frac{x_n}{y_n} = n$

The linear curve passes through the origin indicating that even a mild force can induce a flow. The curve also indicates that the values of η are constant at different shear rates (Fig. 2.5).

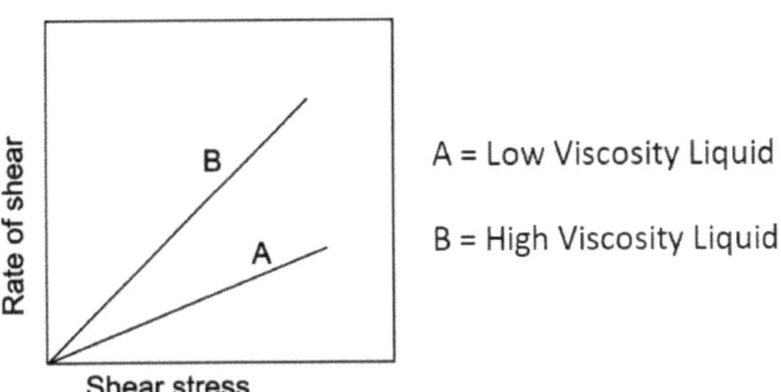

Fig. 2.5 Newtonian flow

Examples of some Newtonian liquids are water, simple organic liquids, solutions containing small solute molecules, dilute suspensions and emulsions.

II. Non-Newtonian systems

A system is said to be non-Newtonian when it shows different η values at different shearing rates at a given temperature. Therefore, the viscosity is often called *apparent* viscosity.

S.No.	Shearing stress	Shear rate	$\eta = \dfrac{Shearing\ stress}{shear\ rate}$
1	x_1	y_1	$\dfrac{x_1}{y_1} = \eta_1$
2	x_2	y_2	$\dfrac{x_2}{y_2} = \eta_2$
3	x_3	y_3	$\dfrac{x_3}{y_3} = \eta_3$
.	.	.	.
.	.	.	.
.	.	.	.
n	x_n	y_n	$\dfrac{x_n}{y_n} = \eta_n$

There are three types of non-Newtonian systems. They are

1. Plastic systems
2. Pseudoplastic systems
3. Dilatant systems

1. Plastic systems

The rheogram of plastic system is shown in (Fig. 2.6).

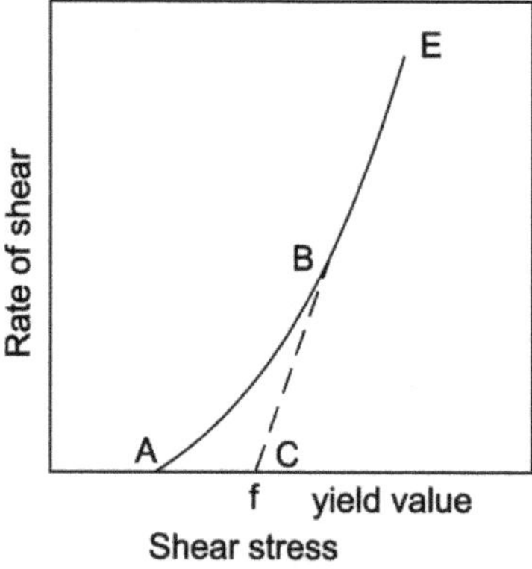

Fig. 2.6 Simple plastic flow

Plastic systems were studied extensively by Bingham and hence, they are called as **Bingham bodies**. In this, the curve is not passing through the origin. It indicates that mild forces cannot induce a flow. The flow is possible only after some shearing stress is exceeded. The shearing stress at *A* is termed as low or minimum or low 'yield value', which induces a flow. The shear stress at the point C is called the *yield value* indicated as *"f"* in the Fig. 2.6. (yield value is an important property of certain pharmaceutical dispersions). At stresses below the yield value *'f'* the substance acts as an elastic material. Then the system is said to behave like a solid for stresses below the yield value. Those substances that exhibit a yield value are, in general, called **Bingham bodies.** It follows that those substances that exhibit no yield value and flows at the smallest shearing stress are termed as fluids. The curve obtained from shear stress *A* to shear stress C is not linear (i.e. the curve *AB*). The slope of the curve gradually increases until the point *B* and it indicates a gradual decrease in the viscosity of the system up to the point *B*. Therefore, the system which shows a gradual decrease in viscosity on increasing the shear stress is called *'shear thinning system'*. In this case, the *apparent plastic viscosity* (U or η_{pl}) is given by

$$\eta_{pl} \text{ or } U = \frac{S - \text{yield value}}{du/dx} \quad \dots (7)$$

Therefore, the η_{pl} viscosity is the viscosity above yield values.

The curve beyond *B* becomes linear (i.e., from B to E) and the system behaves just like Newtonian system there afterwards. The slope of the curve is termed as mobility and its reciprocal as plastic viscosity.

Examples of plastic systems are *ointments, pastes and creams and some disperse systems.*

2. Pseudoplastic systems

The rheogram for pseudoplastic system is given in (Fig. 2.7).

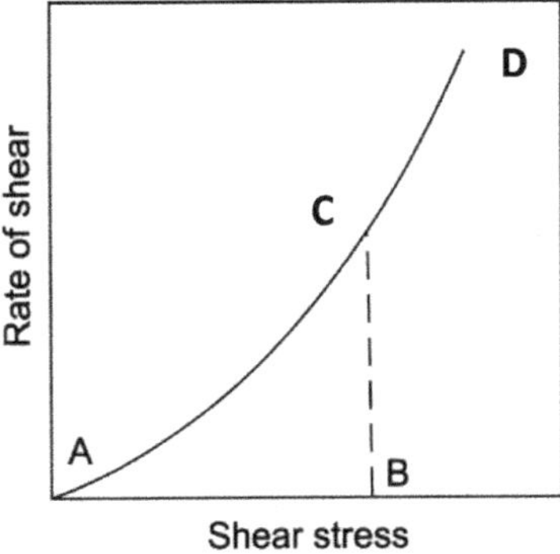

Fig. 2.7

The curve passes through the origin which indicates that mild forces can induce a flow. There is no yield value for this system. The curve obtained from shear stress A to shear stress B is similar to plastic system (i.e., curve AC). Since the system is having both the characters of Newtonian and plastic, it is called pseudoplastic system. This is also a *'shear thinning system'*. In this case, the viscosity is given by the empirical power law.

$$\eta = \frac{S^N}{du/dx} \quad \ldots (8)$$

where the value of N is greater than 1 (For Newtonian system, the value of N is 1). The values of N varies for different pseudoplastic systems. The greater the value of N the more pseudoplastic is the system. The equation (8) can be rearranged and written in logarithmic form as

$$\log \frac{du}{dx} = N \log S - \log \eta$$

Plotting the log of shearing stress ($\log S$) versus the log of rate of shear, $\left(\log \frac{du}{dx}\right)$ a straight line is obtained with a slope of N (Fig. 2.8). However, some pseudoplastic suspending agents do not conform to equation (8)

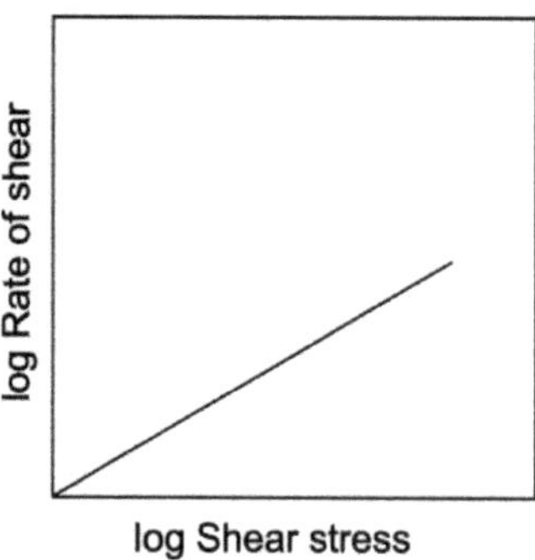

Fig. 2.8 Pseudo-Plastic flow

The curve beyond the point C becomes linear (i.e., from C to D) and the system (Refer Fig 2.7) behaves like Newtonian system there after wards.

To distinguish between plastic and pseudoplastic systems, it is necessary to obtain the flow behavior at low shear rates.

Examples of pseudoplastic system are ***liquid dispersions of tragacanth, sodium alginate and sodium carboxymethyl cellulose.***

3. Dilatant systems

Suspensions with high percentage of dispersed solid particles (i.e., with more than 50% of deflocculated solid dispersed phase) exhibit an increase in resistance to flow with increasing rates of shear. They, in fact, increase in volume (with more void space) when sheared and therefore, termed ***dilatant.*** These Systems show an increase in consistency or viscosity on increasing the shear rate or stress in contrast to 'shear thinning systems' such as pseudoplastic and plastic systems.

The rheogram for dilatant system is given in (Fig. 2.9).

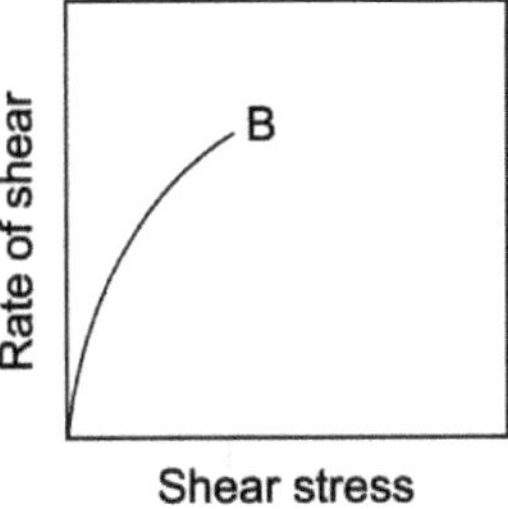

Fig. 2.9

The curve passes through the origin and it indicates that mild forces can induce a flow. The slope of the curve gradually decreases until the point, B. In this case, the viscosity of the system gradually increases and hence this system is called *'Shear thickening system'*. When the stress is removed, a dilatant system returns to its original state of fluidity.

The *apparent* viscosity of a dilatant system is given by the empirical power law.

$$\eta = \frac{S^N}{du/dx} \qquad \text{... (9)}$$

where the value of N is less than 1.

Both the plastic and pseudoplastic systems show *'shear thinning'* properties and the dilatant systems show *'shear thickening'* properties.

Examples of dilatant system are concentrated deflocculated suspension (about 50% or more) and suspensions of starch in water

Mechanism of shear thinning

Plastic system is associated with the presence of aggregates or flocculated particles in the dispersion medium. In pseudoplastic system, the macromolecules align with neighboring molecules resulting in entanglement of molecules entrapping the liquid. In both the cases, there is considerable structural build-up increasing the viscosity of the system. Under the influence of shearing stress in both the systems, there is progressive structural breakdown resulting in decrease in viscosity. Greater amount of breakdown occurs at higher shear rates. Consequently, there is gradual decrease in viscosity. Once the structural breakdown is complete with increasing shear rates, the apparent viscosity becomes constant. i.e., the flow becomes Newtonian.

Mechanism of shear thickening

In contrast to shear thinning system, a shear thickening (or dilatant) system exhibits an increase in viscosity with increasing shear stress or shear rate. In dilatant systems, at rest, the particles are closely packed and so a minimum void space is present. The amount of vehicle is just sufficient to fill the minimum void space and the particles can move relative to one another at low rates of shear. At rest the system is reasonably fluid. As the shear rate is increased, the bulk of the system expands, particles become open packed and the void space within the system increases. The vehicle is now insufficient to fill the expanded void space. As one particle moves with respect to another, there is lot of structural build up with increased void spaces with consequent under-lubrication (i.e., insufficient lubrication) by the medium or vehicle and that leads to increased viscosity. Eventually the fluid system becomes a firm paste-like. Hence processing of dilatant systems in a mixer such as colloid mill leads to overloading and damaging the processing equipment especially at high shear rates

The following figure (Fig 2.10) shows dilatant system at rest and at high shear rates.

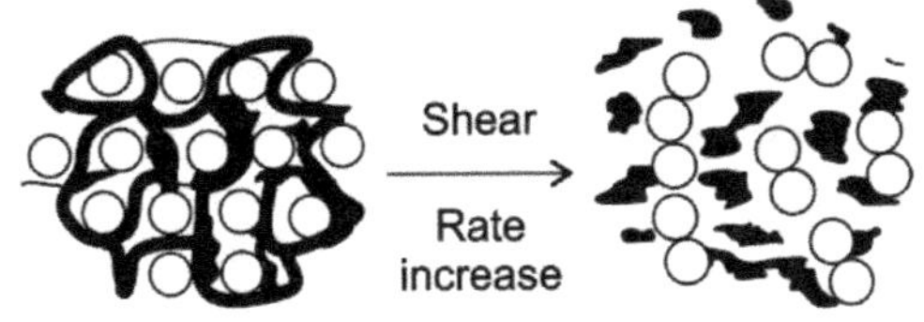

Dilatant system at rest	Dilatant system at high shear rate
Particles closely packed	Particles open packed
Less void space	More void space
Vehicle sufficient to fill the void space	Vehicle not sufficient to fill the void space
Less viscous and pourable	More viscous and non-pourable

Thixotropy

In the case of Newtonian systems, a curve which may be called up-curve is obtained with increase in shear rate. If the rate of shear is reduced after the desired maximum rate has been reached, a down-curve may be obtained. This down-curve and up-curve would be identical and superimposable. Whereas in shear-thinning system (i.e., in non-Newtonian systems), the down-curve can be displaced with respect to the up-curve. This indicates that the material has a different (especially lower) consistency at anyone rate of shear on the down-curve. It may be assumed tacitly that the system adapts itself to changing shear instantaneously. It may also be assumed that the structural build-up may not follow the same route of the structural break-up for its return to its original state i.e., structural build-up will not be the exact inverse copy for the structural break-up) because of changing rate of shear and the time of shear. The plastic and pseudoplastic systems at a given temperature, change their viscosities at varying shearing stresses.

By gradually increasing the shearing stress on plastic or pseudoplastic systems, the apparent viscosity gradually decreases as a result of progressive breakdown of structure in the liquid medium at a given temperature. After removing the shearing stress, the viscosity is regained due to slow rebuilding of structure by Brownian motion but not immediately but after some time lag. Consider the conversion of gel to sol and then sol to gel after removing the stress applied.

$$\text{Gel} \underset{\text{removing shear sterss}}{\overset{\text{applying shear stress}}{\rightleftharpoons}} \text{Sol}$$

The conversion of sol to gel is not instantaneous but requires some time lag indicating its time-dependency.

Plastic and pseudoplastic systems will change their viscosities gradually with respect to time even if a constant shearing stress is applied. They show a lower consistency or viscosity at any one shear rate on the down-curve than it had on the up-curve. It indicates that the build-up of structure does not take place immediately to regain its original consistency when the stress is removed or reduced. This phenomenon, called thixotropy, may now be defined as ***a reversible isothermal transition from gel to sol with a comparatively slow recovery from sol to gel on standing or at rest.*** In consistent with this definition, thixotropy can be applied only to shear-thinning systems.

A rheogram can be obtained for a shear thinning systems by plotting the rate of shear at various shear stresses. The curve is called `up curve'. By reducing the shearing stress gradually on the above system, a `down-curve' is obtained. Both the `up curve' and `down curve' are not super-imposable. The down curve is shifted to left side. This means the flow property of the system is not the same before and after the initial determination. Hence the viscosity of the sample depends upon its previous history. Therefore, the viscosities of the `down curve' are lower than the viscosities of the `up curve'. As a result, the `down curve' is shifted to the left side of the `up curve' in the rheogram (Fig. 2.11).

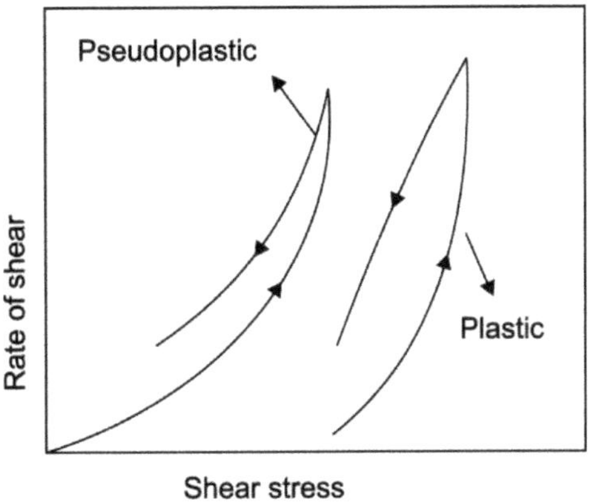

Fig. 2.11 Thixotropy in plastic and pseudoplastic systems

Rheograms obtained with shear-thinning systems are, thus, highly dependent on the rate at which shear is increased or decreased and the length of time the system is subjected to any one rate of shear. Simply saying, it depends on the previous history of the sample taken. The loop between the `up curve' and the `down curve' is called `hysteresis loop'. The area of the loop indicates the extent of structural breakdown.

An example of the system showing thixotropy is bentonite gel. Even the curd obtained from milk can be considered as a thixotropic material.

Bulges and sours

Some dispersions may yield complex hysteresis loop. Though it is not so important, it may need a mention about. For example, a 10 to 15% by weight of aqueous bentonite gel yields a hysteresis loop with a characteristic bulge in the up-curve as shown in the Fig. 2.12. It is assumed to be due to the swelling of bentonite resulting from the crystalline plates of bentonite forming a "house of cards structure"

It is reported that in still more structured system such as procaine penicillin gel, the bulge develops into a spur-like protrusion demonstrating a high yield or spur value as shown in Fig. 2.13. The spur value γ represents a sharp of structural breakdown at low shear stress. It was found gels having definite spur values were very thixotropic, forming intramuscular depots upon injection. Such depots afford prolonged blood levels of the drug.

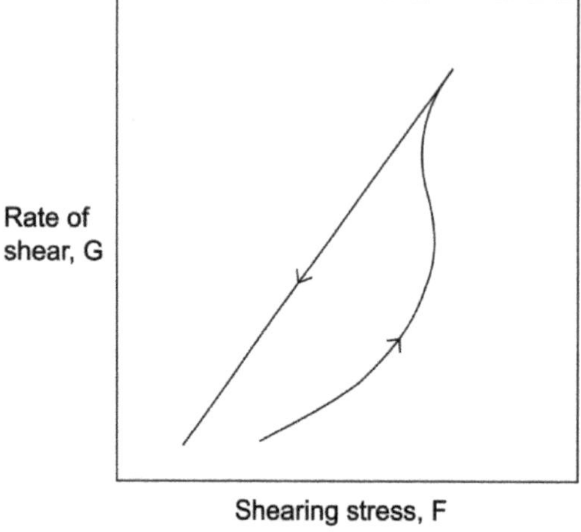

Fig. 2.12 Rheogram of a thixotropic material showing a bulge in the hysteresis loop

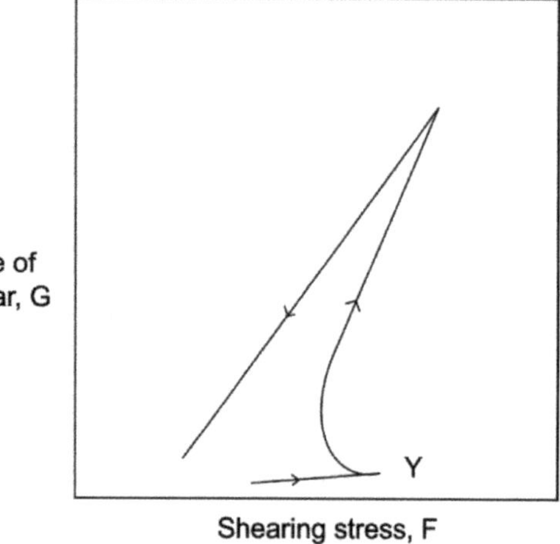

Fig. 2.13 Rheogram of a thixotropic material showing a spur value Y in the hysteresis loop

Negative thixotropy and rheopecy

Certain thixotropic materials show a phenomenon called *negative thixotropy* or *anti-thixotropy*. A thixotropic system such as magnesia magma exhibits an increase rather than a decrease in viscosity on the down curve. The magma which showed normal thixotropy below the shear rates of 30 per second, showed negative thixotropy at shear rates greater than 30 per second. In this the down curve was shifted to right side indicating an increase in viscosity.

The rebuilding of the broken structure after it has been subjected to certain shear rates takes some more time to regain its original consistency. In this case the restoration by Brownian motion is slow if the suspensions or solutions are viscous. However, in such cases gentle agitation or moderate and rhythmic vibration may speed up the rebuilding of the structure. Low shear rates thus hasten the process of regaining the initial high apparent viscosity or the onset of gelation in thixotropic sols. If the sheared dispersion of bentonite in a beaker is subjected to gentle vibration or rotation, the rebuilding of the 'house of cards' is speeded up. This material's recovery of some of its pre-sheared viscosity at a faster rate when it is gently sheared, compared to when it allowed to stand, is called *rheopecy*.

Determination of Flow Properties

For Newtonian systems, the shear rate is directly proportional to the shearing stress and hence it is enough to find a single rate of shear for a shearing stress (i.e., one point determination.) The point obtained for this value in the graph may be extrapolated to the origin i.e., a line passing through the point and origin may be drawn. The line gives a complete rheogram. For non-Newtonian systems, one point determination is useless and hence a multi-point determination should be undertaken. i.e., a number of rates of shear must be obtained at different shearing stresses to obtain a complete rheogram for plastic, pseudoplastic and dilatant systems.

The different instruments used for the determination of flow properties are

1. Ostwalds Viscometer
2. Ubbelohde Suspended Level Viscometer
3. Falling Sphere Viscometer
4. Cup and Bob Viscometer
5. Cone and Plate Viscometer.

Of these five viscometers, the first three viscometers are used for the determination of Newtonian flow and the last two are used for the determination of both Newtonian and non-Newtonian flows.

1. Ostwald's Viscometer

It is also called capillary viscometer. The apparatus (Fig. 2.14) consists of a `$U$' tube, the left arm of the tube has a `bulging' at its lower part and there is a marking `$A$' above this bulb. The right arm of the tube also has a `bulging' at the upper part and just below this bulb is a capillary tube as shown in the figure. There are two markings B and C above and below the bulb of the right arm.

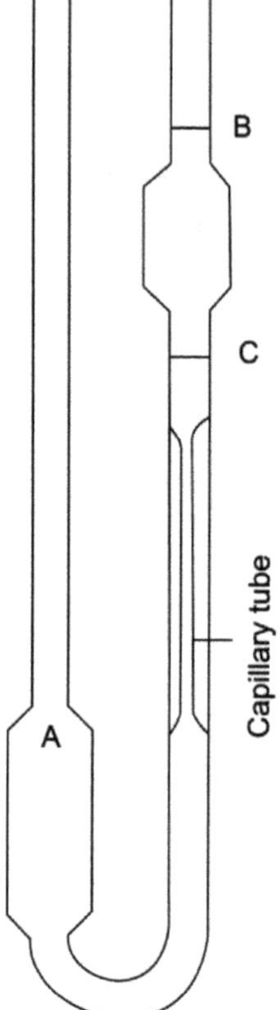

Fig. 2.14 Ostwald's Viscometer

The liquid is poured into the apparatus through the left arm up to the mark *A*. The liquid is then sucked into the right arm slightly above the point *B* and the left arm is closed with the thumb to keep the liquid without dropping down. The apparatus is clamped vertically and the thumb is removed so as to allow the liquid to fall through the capillary under gravity. The time taken for the liquid level to drop down from the point *B* to *C* is noted. The room temperature is also noted. As per Poisuille's equation.

$$\eta = \frac{\pi}{8}\frac{pr^4t}{Vl} = \frac{\pi}{8}\frac{hdgr^4t}{Vl} \qquad \ldots (10)$$

$$\eta = ctd$$

where c is instrument constant

The instrument constant is usually supplied along with the instrument by the manufacturer. By knowing the value of the time t to flow from the mark B to C and the density of the liquid d, the absolute viscosity of the liquid can be found out.

The relative viscosity of the liquid with respect to water can be found out as follows.

The experiment is first undertaken for water as described above with the instrument. After cleaning and drying the instrument, the experiment is carried out with the liquid whose relative viscosity is to be found out.

$$\frac{\eta_l}{\eta_w} = \frac{ct_l d_l}{ct_w d_w} = \frac{t_l d_l}{t_w d_w} \quad \text{... (12)}$$

The viscosity of water η_w at a given temperature (may be room temperature) is found out. Then t_l, d_l, t_w, and d_w are determined. From these values, the relative viscosity of the liquid with respect to water can be found out. The relative viscosity of the liquid may be converted to absolute viscosity by multiplying the relative viscosity with the absolute viscosity of water. The viscosities of the liquid can be found out at different temperatures by keeping the instrument in a thermostat.

Sometimes the viscosity of the liquid is expressed as *kinematic* viscosity

$$v = \frac{\eta}{\rho} = \frac{\text{absolute viscosity}}{\text{density of the liquid}} \quad \text{... (13)}$$

Experimental precautions

1. Streamline flow must occur in the capillary
2. Unnecessary long flow time should be avoided.
3. There should not be any air bubble.
4. The instrument should be thoroughly cleaned and dried for each liquid.
5. Adequate temperature control should be ensured.
6. Correction may be made for surface tension which tends to raise or lower the meniscus of the liquid in the tube.

The disadvantage with the Ostwald's viscometer is that for relative viscosity determination, volume of liquid put into the apparatus should be constant so as to get correct reproducible result.

To avoid the above difficulties, Ubbelohde viscometer is used.

2. Ubbelohde viscomenter

It is a modified Ostwald's viscometer and in this another vertical tube (third arm) is attached to the bulb below the capillary part of the right arm parallel to `U' tube as shown in (Fig. 2.15).

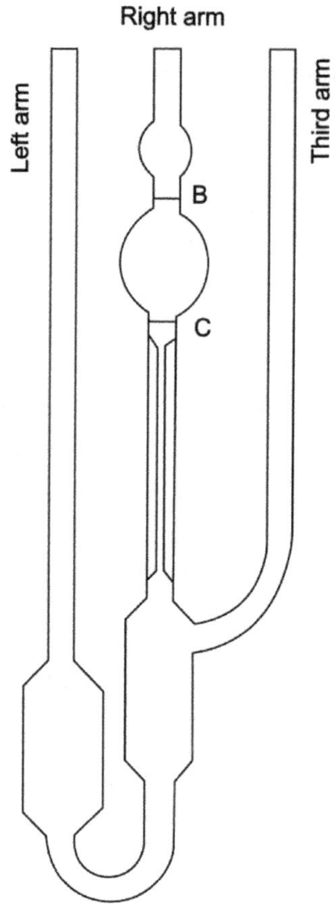

Fig. 2.15 Ubbelohde viscometer

A volume of liquid just sufficient to fill the bulb in the left arm is poured. By closing the left arm and the third arm with the thumbs, the liquid is sucked into the right arm (i.e. central tube) upto a level just above the point B. The central arm is now closed with the thumb after removing the thumbs from the other two arms and that keeps the level of the liquid just above the mark B. As the liquid below the capillary tube is ventilated down by the third arm, the volume of liquid in the right arm (central tube) remains constant. The rest of the experiment is similar to as described under Ostwald's viscometer.

3. Falling sphere viscometer (Hoeppler falling ball viscometer)

As per Stoke's law, a body falling through a viscous medium, experiences a resistance or viscous drag that opposes the motion of the body. When the body falls through a liquid under the influence of gravity during which acceleration of the motion occurs at the initial period but when the gravitational force (acceleration) is balanced by the viscous drag, the body falls down at a uniform terminal velocity which can be determined in the falling sphere viscometer.

Viscous drag on the sphere = force responsible for downward motion due to gravity.

$$3\pi \ \eta du = \frac{\pi}{6} \ d^3 g \ (\rho_s - \rho_l) \qquad \text{... (14)}$$

where η = coefficient of viscosity

d = diameter of the sphere

g = acceleration due to gravity

u = terminal velocity

ρ_s = density of the sphere

ρ_l = density of the liquid

Rearranging the above equation

$$\eta = \frac{d^2 g \ (\rho_s - \rho_l)}{18u} \qquad \text{... (15)}$$

The diameter of the sphere may be obtained by using vernier caliper. ρ_l (density of the liquid) is determined using specific gravity bottle and the terminal velocity (u) by using the falling sphere viscometer and from these values the viscosity of the liquid may be calculated.

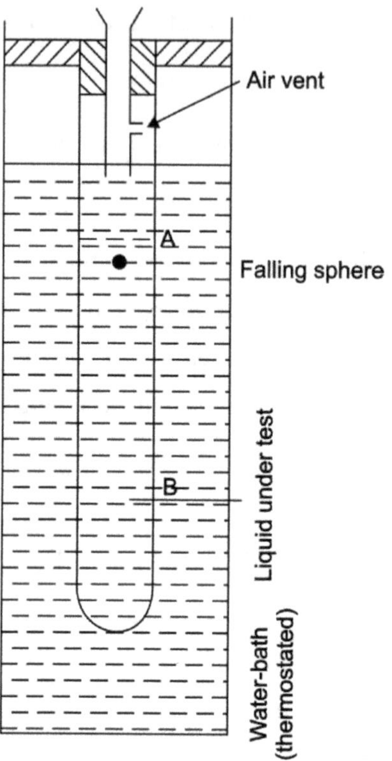

Fig. 2.16 Falling sphere viscometer

The apparatus (Fig. 2.16) consists of a tube having two markings A and B marked on the outer surface of the tube. The tube is filled with the liquid whose viscosity is to be determined. The tube is clamped vertically inside a constant temperature bath. Sufficient time is allowed to get all the air bubbles removed and the whole set up to attain the equilibrium temperature. A steel sphere (ball) is cleaned and allowed to reach the same temperature as that of the experiment by keeping in a thermostat. There is a guide tube on the fall tube through which the ball is allowed to fall and a hole in the guide tube prevents any airlock. The time `$t'$ taken for the sphere to fall from $A$ to $B$ is noted. The terminal velocity is the ratio of the distance between the two markings $A$ and $B$ and the time `t'. By substituting all the values in the equation, the coefficient of the viscosity of the liquid is calculated.

The equation is given assuming that the sphere is falling through a medium of infinite dimension. But in the experiment the liquid is contained in a cylinder. A correction factor (F) is introduced to nullify the effect of wall on the fall of the sphere.

$$F = 1 - \frac{2.104d}{D} + 2.09\frac{d^3}{D^3} \quad \text{... (16)}$$

where d = diameter of the sphere

D = diameter of the tube

and the corrected viscosity = $\eta \times F$

The instrument can be used over a range of 0.5 to 200,000 poise. For best results, the ball (density) should be such that it takes not less than 30 seconds to fall from mark A to B.

(***Red Wood Viscometer:*** It consists of a cylinder having an outlet at its bottom with a valve. Two sizes are available called No.1 and No.2. The specifications are detailed in British Pharmacopoeia. The liquid is filled up to the mark made in the cylinder. The valve is fully opened and the time taken for the liquid to drain out fully is reported as Redwood seconds. Thus, it is an empirical instrument.)

4. Rotational viscometer

In rotational viscometers a solid rotating body is immersed or suspended in a liquid/semi solid (whose viscosity is to be measured) and is subjected to a retarding force due to the viscous drag which is proportional to the viscosity of the liquid. The advantages of rotational viscometers are:

(a) it is possible to vary the shear rate over a wide range of values and
(b) measurements can be made continuously for extended periods at a given shear rate or shear stress.

Therefore, the rotational viscometer, with accurate temperature control, are useful for measuring the time dependency as well as shear dependency of the viscosities of non-Newtonian systems. The rotational viscometers are

1. Concentric cylinder viscometer (or co-axial cylinder viscometer or cup and bob viscometers)
2. cone and plate viscometers.

Cup and Bob viscometer

The cup and bob viscometer (Fig. 2.17) consists of an outer cylinder *A*, (cup) which acts as a container for the liquid, and can be rotated at different speeds (different shearing stresses). An inner cylinder *B* (bob) is suspended freely by a torsion wire. Rotation of the outer cylinder A produces movements within the liquid in the gap separating the two cylinders and as a result the torque (indicating rate of shear) produced is transmitted to the inner cylinder *B*. This torque (*T*) is measured in terms of angular deflection θ of a pointer which moves on a scale.

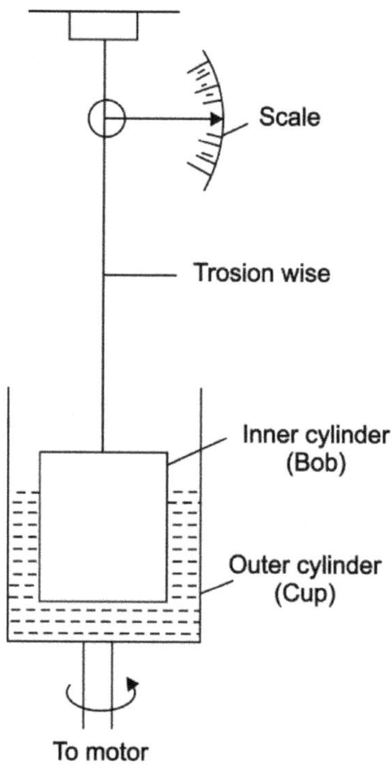

Fig. 2.17 Concentric cylinder viscometer (coutte type)

If a steady laminar flow occurs within the liquid, the viscosity is calculated as follows:

$$\eta = \frac{T_o\left(\frac{1}{r_1^2} - \frac{1}{r_2^2}\right)}{4\pi h\omega} \qquad \dots (17)$$

Where, T_o = torque in dynes cm.

r_1 and r_2 = radii of the inner and outer cylinders

h = height of the inner cylinder surrounded by the liquid.

ω = angular velocity of the outer cylinder

There are two types of viscometers

(a) *Couette type viscometer:* The cup is revolved. The viscous drag on the bob produced by the liquid results in a torque which is proportional to viscosity e.g: *Mac Machael viscometer.*

(b) *Searle type viscometer:* It involves the principle of rotating the bob instead of the cup. e.g.: ***Stromer viscometer*** (Fig.2.18). For systems of viscosity more than 20 centipoise, it may be used. In this the cup is placed in a thermostat (constant temperature bath) on a stand and the bob is suspended into it. Both the cup and bob are allowed to reach the equilibrium temperature. The bob can be rotated by placing weight on a hanger through a winding pool which is attached to a hanger through a pulley. The number of revolutions of the bob can be counted with the help of a revolution counter. The data are converted to rpm. The weight is increased and the whole procedure is similar to the above.

The rpm value can be converted to actual shear rates. The weight aided can be transposed into the units of shear stress, dynes/cm^2

Formula for shear rate = k_g.n where n is adjustable speed i.e. rpm and k_g = shear rate factor

Formula for shear stress = $K_F S$. Where, S is dial reading and K_F, shear stress factor.

A rheogram can be obtained by plotting rpm versus the weight added. Making use of appropriate constants, rpm values are converted to actual shear rates (sec^{-1}) and the weights added into the units of shear (dynes cm^{-2}) In this case, the viscosity is calculated as follows

$$\eta = K_v \frac{w}{v} \quad \text{... (18)}$$

where w = weight in grams

v = rpm generated due to w

K_v = instrument constant which can be determined by analysing an oil of known viscosity using the instrument.

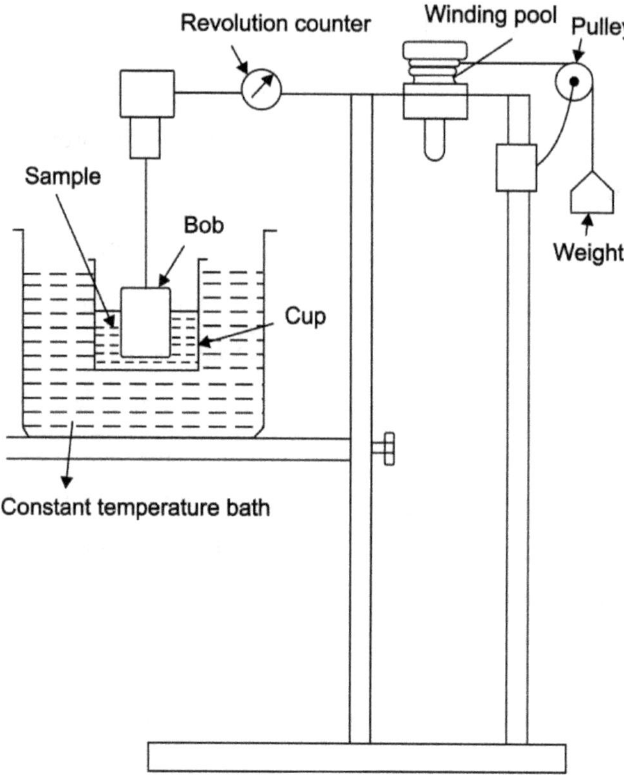

Fig. 2.18 Stromer Viscometer (Searle type)

The plastic viscosity may be calculated using the formula, when Stromer viscometer is used.

$$U = K_v \frac{W - W_f}{V} \quad \text{... (19)}$$

where W_f yield value intercept in grams.

The yield value of a Bingham body (f) (plastic system) is given by the expression.

$$f = K_f \times W_f \quad \text{... (20)}$$

Where

$$K_f = K_v \times \frac{2\pi}{60} \times \frac{1}{2.303 \log\left(\frac{R_2}{R_1}\right)} \quad \text{... (21)}$$

where R_2 = radius of the cup

R_1 = radius of the bob

Disadvantages of cup and bob viscometer

1. If the gap between the cup and bob is larger, there will be no uniform rate of shear.
2. Frictional heating may develop at higher rates of shear and hence a constant temperature bath is used to offset the temperature effect on viscosity of the liquid.
3. Filling and cleaning are often difficult.
4. The instrument requires more sample.
5. *Plug flow development:* In the cup and bob viscometer there is a variable shear stress within the sample across the gap between the cup and bob. This variation is mainly dependent upon the gap. In Searle type viscometer, the bob is rotated and the cup is stationary. For the bob to be rotated, the shearing stress should necessarily be higher than the yield value. It may happen so, for a certain shearing stress of the bob, (though it is sufficiently high to exceed the yield value) the shearing stress developed at the inner surface of the cup may be less than the yield value. In such a situation, the material at the inner surface of the cup remains as a solid plug without any flow. This phenomenon is plug flow. Chances of plug flow can be minimized by reducing the gap between the cup and bob. For that a bob as large as possible may be used. Laminar flow (rather than plug flow) of the system can be expected only when the shear stress at the wall of the cup exceeds the yield value).

Plug flow may be important when pastes and concentrated suspensions flow out of the container through an orifice. For example, in the case of tooth paste obtained from its container, the paste experiences a higher shear stress when pressed at the circumference of the tube aperture. As a result, the consistency drops at the points of stress and this facilitates extrusion of the paste in the core as a plug. However, this phenomenon is not desirable in obtaining rheograms of plastic systems with cup and bob viscometer.

Cone and plate viscometer

In cone and plate viscometer, all the disadvantages mentioned under cup and bob viscometer are overcome.

The cone and plate viscometer (Fig. 2.19) essentially consists of a smooth plate and a cone. During operation, the sample is placed at the center of the plate, which is then slowly raised so that the tip of the cone comes in contact with the sample. At this position, the cone to plate angle is ordinarily less than 1°C. The sample is sheared in the narrow gap between the plate and the cone when the plate is driven by a variable speed motor. The torque transmitted through the sample to the cone is measured. The viscosity is given by

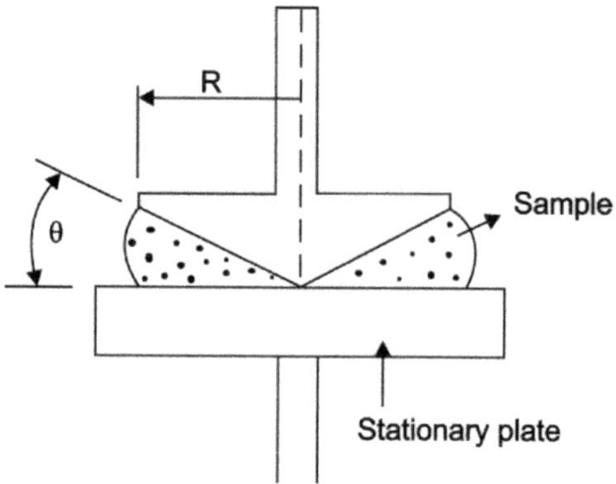

Fig. 2.19 Cone and plate viscometer

$$\eta = \frac{3A/2\pi R^3}{B/Q} \qquad \text{... (22)}$$

where A = torque on the cone

R = radius of the cone

B = radial velocity of the plate

Q = angle between the cone and the plate and is less than $\pi/360$ radians

Advantages:

1. Rate of shear is constant throughout the sample and hence no chance for plug flow.
2. Cleaning is easy and requires less time.
3. Temperature stabilization is also good.
4. It needs vary little sample for the study. That is a sample volume of 0.1 to 0.2 ml will do.
5. Rates of shear can be increased or decreased in a predetermined and reproducible manner.
6. This serves as a valuable aid for the determination of hysteresis loop obtained in thixotropic systems and also in determining thixotropic coefficient.

Commercial Viscometers

1. Ferranti - Portable viscometer
2. Brookfield viscometer
3. Ferranti - Shirley cone and plate viscometer
4. Extrusion viscometer

1. Ferranti - Portable viscometer (for bulk liquids)

In this the rotating outer cylinder is inverted and immersed in the liquid. The inner cylinder is attached to a pointer on a scale through a torque spring which is beryllium copper spring. (Fig. 2.20) There is a guard ring shown in Fig. 2.20.

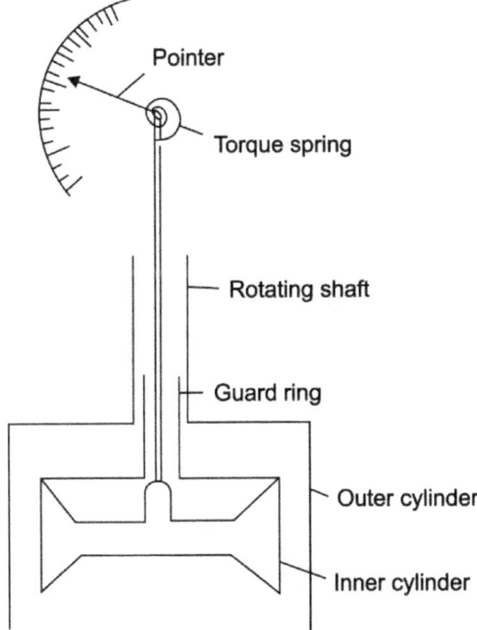

Fig. 2.20 Ferranti portable viscometer

The outer cylinder is driven by a synchronous motor with a three to five speed gear box. The gear box can provide a range of 1 rev/min. up to 300 rev/min. The mean shear rates vary from 930 to 0.15 sec^{-1}. Amount of sample required is usually about 100 ml. For a given rpm (rate of shear) and the angle of deflection (shearing stress), the viscosity may be read directly from the literature table supplied by the manufacturer.

2. Brookfield viscometer

It is used as a comparative instrument (Fig. 2.21) since it does not provide results in terms of absolute shear. A bob is immersed in the sample liquid. The bob carries a rotating spindle which is driven through a calibrated beryllium copper spring which in turn is mounted on a motor shaft. The spindle is also attached to a pointer which gives the displacement of the spindle due to viscous drag of the sample. Since both the pointer and the scale revolve, the readings are complicated. However, it is possible to clamp the pointer. In this viscosity changes cannot be followed while increasing the shearing stress and hence it is used for comparing the apparent viscosities of non-Newtonian systems.

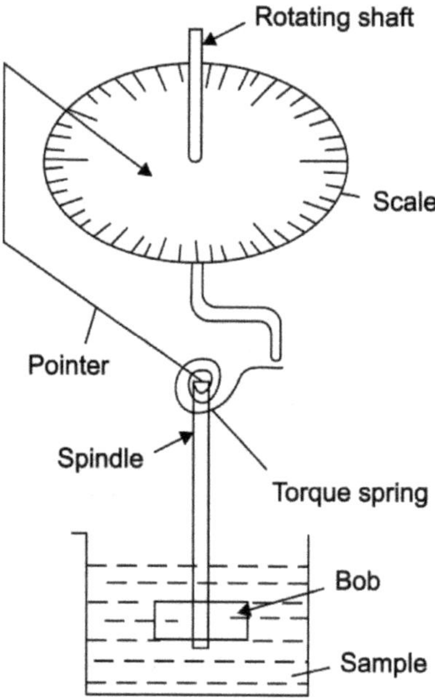

Fig. 2.21 Brookfield Viscometer

3. Ferranti - Shirley cone and plate viscometer

It is very popularly used to study the change of flow properties of a rheological system continuously by varying the shear rates and to study thixotropy.

This viscometer (Fig. 2.22) consists of a stationary flat plate and a rotating cone. The usual plate to cone angle is about 0.3° to 4° so that only small samples (0.1 to 0.2 ml) are required. The plate is maintained at a constant temperature.

The rate of shear for small angles is constant and is given by

$$\frac{A}{B} \quad \text{... (23)}$$

where A = rotation (rad/sec)

B = cone angle (rad)

The cone is driven by a variable speed motor and the rate of shear is capable of being varied over a wide range from 0 to 18000 sec^{-1}. A torsion spring is interposed between the cone (i.e., the driving shaft of the cone) and the driving shaft in order to measure the shearing stress on a galvanometer connected to a potentiometer circuit.

It is possible to obtain recording of shear rates and shearing stresses simultaneously. This enables to obtain flow curves automatically on an $x - y$ recorder.

A rheological system is taken in between the cone and the plate. The rate of shear is varied continuously and the corresponding shearing stresses are recorded simultaneously on $x - y$ recorder. From the rheograms obtained, one can make out whether the system is Newtonian, plastic, pseudoplastic or dilatant.

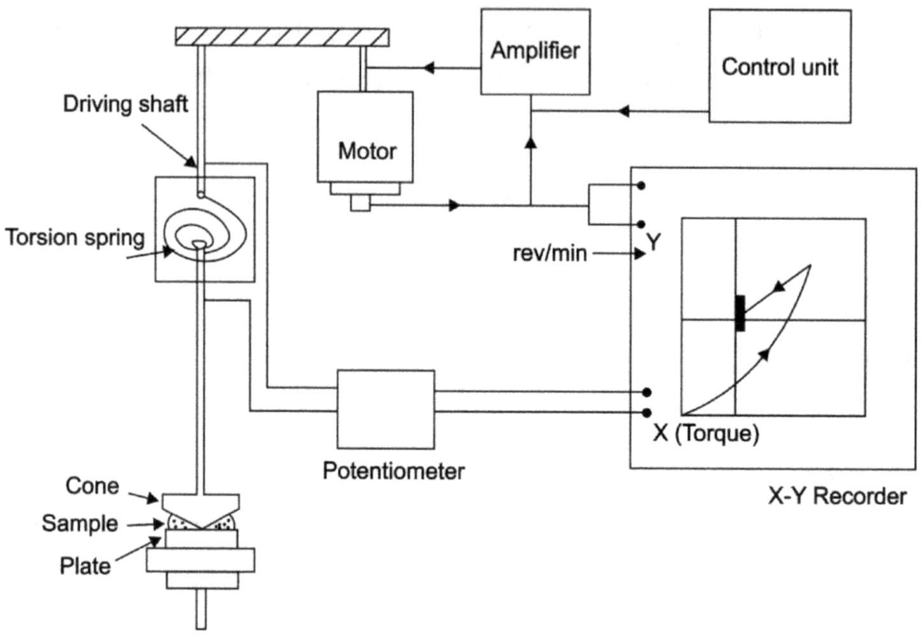

Fig. 2.22 Ferranti-shirely cone and plate viscometer

For thixotropic studies, a sample is placed in between the cone and plate in the instrument. The rate of shear is gradually increased and the corresponding shear stresses are recorded simultaneously on the $x - y$ recorder to get the `up-curve'. Then the rate of shear is gradually decreased in the sample and the corresponding shearing stresses are recorded simultaneously on the $x - y$ recorder to obtain the `down curve'. Thus, it is possible to demonstrate the time-dependent effect of stresses on rheological systems as well as how the previous history of the sample alters its physical properties.

4. Extrusion viscometer

It is suitable for butter and semisolid preparations. It consists of a simple cylinder 4 cm long and 1.25 cm in diameter with a circular orifice. Inside the cylinder is a plunger which could be moved at a uniform speed.

A sample of any ointment or paste or cream which has got consumer acceptability is kept in the cylinder. The thrust just required to extrude the material is recorded. Whether the sample of ointment or paste or cream is having the same thrust for the subsequent batches are tested. Any non-homogeneity due to substandard material, agglomerate of particles or air bubble will be indicated by the fluctuation in the recorded thrust.

Deformation of solids

When a solid body is subjected to opposing forces on its opposite sides, there is a finite change in its geometry or shape depending upon the nature of applied forces or load. The relative amount of deformation produced by such forces is a dimensionless quantity called *strain*. The various types of strains may be tensile strain, compression strain and shear strain. Consider a solid of definite geometry is compressed by forces acting on its opposite sides to cause a reduction in length of ΔH. if the initial length before the application of force is H_o (Fig. 2.23), the compression strain, Z may be given by the equation

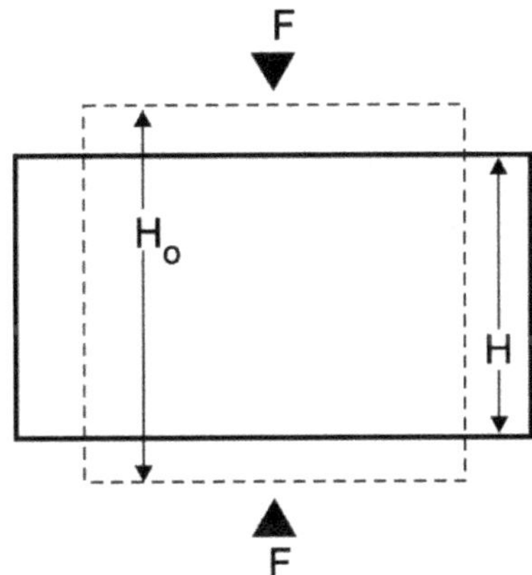

Fig. 2.23

$$Z = \frac{\Delta H}{H_o}$$

The ratio of the force, F required to produce the strain to the area, A over which it acts is called thr stress, σ and is given by

$$\sigma = \frac{F}{A}$$

Stress is the force or load applied on solid at a particular area or angle and strain is the effect produced.

Deformation of solids may comprise two components – elastic deformation and plastic deformation.

Elastic deformation

When an external mechanical force is applied to a mass of powder of certain volume contained in a container, the powder particles may repack and this repacking leads to some internal volume reduction. When this repacking resulting in volume reduction becomes more difficult, there may be some type of powder particle deformation on further compression. This powder particle deformation results mainly from the change in intermolecular spacing. This intermolecular spacing is reversible to a large extent on on removal of the load. In otherwords, there is spontaneous reversibility. The solid particles behave like rubber and hence the deformation is said to be elastic. All solids undergo some elastic deformation when subjected to external forces not exceeding the elastic limit. Thus, in the initial stage of stress or applied pressure the deformation of solid material will be elastic. Once the applied load is released or removed, the material will return to its original shape.

Mostly, a solid material, under the initial stages of applied pressure, will be deformed elastically and a change in the shape of the solid material caused by the applied pressure becomes completely reversible and the material will return to its original shape on release of the pressure. The stress-strain relationship for a specimen of solid material is described by ***Hooke's law.*** For an ideal elastic solid, Hooke's law states that the strain is directly proportional to the applied pressure (or stress) within the elastic limit of the material and can be given by,

$$\sigma = E \,.\, \epsilon$$

Where σ = applied pressure or stress

E = Young's modulus of elasticity and it is a measure of the stiffness, hardness, or resistance to elongation.

ϵ = strain

The strain can be given by $\epsilon = \frac{l - l_o}{l_o}$

Where, l_o = initial length and l = final length. Young's modulus,

The elastic strain results from a change in the intermolecular spacing and for a small deformation. It is reversible. As long as the elastic limit is not exceeded, the material shows elastic deformation. If the elastic limit is exceeded, the deformation of the material becomes irreversible. In pharmaceutical materials such as acetyl salicylic acid and microcrystalline cellulose, elastic deformation assumes the dominant mechanism of compression even within the range of maximum forces normally encountered in practice.

Plastic deformation

In other groups of powdered solids, an elastic limit or yield point is reached and application of load above this limit results in deformation not immediately reversible on removal of applied pressure. In these cases, bulk volume reduction results from plastic deformation and/or viscous flow of the particles. Squeezing of particles into the remaining void space represents the viscous flow of particles. Such a mechanism predominates in materials in which the shear strength (or stress) is less than the breaking strength. When the shear strength is greater the particles may be preferentially fractured or broken. The smaller particles may then fill up any adjacent void or air spaces. Such a fracture is termed brittle fracture. There may also be ductile fracture which is characterized by extensive plastic deformation followed by fracture. All the deformation effects may be accompanied by breaking and formation of new bonds between the particles resulting in consolidation as the new surfaces are pressed together.

Thus, plastic deformation is the permanent change in the shape of the solid material due to applied stress. Plastic deformation depends entirely on crystal defects such as dislocation, grain boundaries and slip planes within the crystals and this in turn is influenced by the rate of crystallization, particle size, the presence of impurities, and the type of crystallization solvent used. The following stress-strain curve (Fig. 2.24) depicts elastic and plastic deformation.

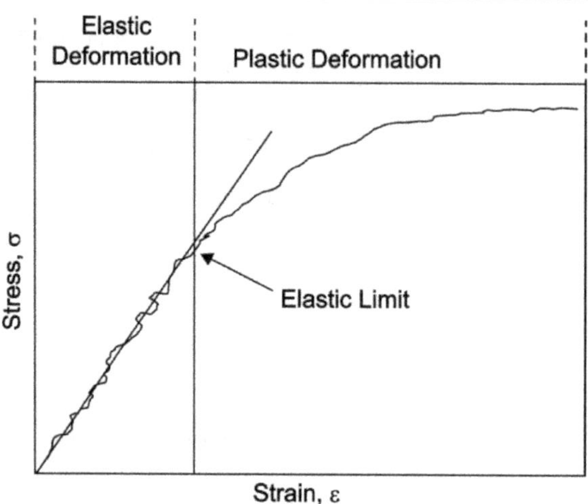

Fig. 2.24 Stress-strain curve showing elastic and plastic deformation regions

Plastic deformation assumes importance because; the plastic deformation permits pharmaceutical excipients and drugs to establish large areas of contact during compaction which assures strong tablets ensuring less friability also.

The student must understand, at this juncture, that when a bed of powder is subjected to compression forces, there is initial repacking followed by elastic and plastic deformation. All these three processes lead to volume reduction resulting in a compact mass of powder or pack, say tablet.

This reduction in volume, which is actually the reduction in void space amoung powder particles, leads to changes in density of the powder pack. Therefore, in tablet compression, an important concept is relative density. The relative density, D, of a (powder) material is given by

$$D = \rho / \rho_o$$

Where ρ = density of the powder material pack in g/cm^3

ρ_o = true density (or absolute density) of powder material in g/cm^3

True density can be defined as the density of the powder material in the absence of pores within it. It means the powder pack contains absolutely no void spaces between particles.

In tablet compression, the relative density has a maximum value of 1.0 and this occurs when all the void space is compressed out of the compressed powder and only solid material (i.e. the tablet) with no pores remains. Attainment of a relative density value of 1.0 is virtually impossible. Usually, relative density values in pharmaceutical tablets may range from 0.4 to 0.95 from loose powder to highly compressed tablets.

Almost all tablets may have some porous structure. The typical density for tablets may vary from 0.7 to 0.95. It means 30% to 10% of tablet volume consists of pores. The relation between relative density and porosity is given by

$$\epsilon = 1 - D$$

Where ϵ = porosity and D = relative density

Heckle equation which relates the applied pressure to porosity, is based on the assumption that void space decrease follows first order process. The Heckel equation is

$$\frac{dD}{dP} = K.(1 - D)$$

Where $\frac{dD}{dP}$ = change in density (hence in porosity) with increase in applied pressure or load

K = slope and is a measure of plasticity. A greater slope indicates greater plasticity

of the material.

A = related to the initial repacking when pressure is zero.

Integrating the above equation, we can get

$$ln\frac{1}{1-D} = K.P + A$$

A Heckel plot can be obtained by plotting $ln1/1 - D$ versus *P*. Such a plot may consist of two regions – an initial non-linear region followed by a linear region. It is to be understood that the Heckel equation does not apply to non-linear portion and it reflects the initial stage of consolidation where significant rearrangement takes place. The terminal portion of the plot is linear which obeys the Heckel equation indicating the deformation properties. The following Heckel plots for three different materials show different terminal slops indicating different deformation properties.

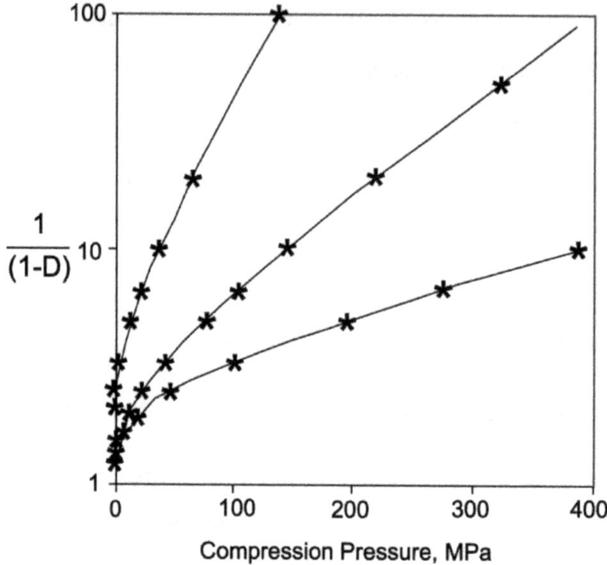

Fig. 2.25 Heckel plot of three pharmaceutical agents

3. COARSE DISPERSIONS

Introduction

As already mentioned under colloidal dispersions, coarse dispersions are the third type of dispersions which are to be discussed in suspensions and emulsions in this chapter. The study of these systems is of pharmaceutical importance especially the suspensions which paves a way to formulate insoluble as well as bitter tasting drugs into liquid dosage forms. Some highly bitter tasting drugs can be converted to an insoluble form by chemical modification and then formulated as suspensions.

Emulsions also offer a way to mask the obnoxious smell of drugs (especially the oils) facilitating the oral route of administration of drugs in liquid form. Another advantage of these coarse dispersions (suspensions and emulsions) is better absorption because of increase in surface area.

1. SUSPENSIONS

A suspension is a heterogeneous (biphasic) system consisting of a solid phase in a liquid phase. The solid phase is subdivided into small particles and dispersed in the liquid medium in which the solid is insoluble or sparingly (or slightly) soluble. Suspensions being coarse dispersions, the size of the greater number of particles may exceed 0.1 μ.

A pharmaceutical suspension may be defined as a coarse dispersion of finely subdivided insoluble solid drug suspended with suitable suspending agents in a suitable liquid (usually aqueous) medium. A suspension may be for internal, external or parenteral use.

Suspensions for oral administration is a better means of administration than of solid dosage forms such as tablets and capsules especially when swallowing is difficult. Thus, they prove more useful for administering for infants and old patients. As suspensions contain subdivided solid particles, surface area is large and this is taken advantage of for drugs which are adsorptives or antacids. Examples may be kaolin, magnesium trisilicate suspensions etc. Often drugs which are bitter in soluble form are administered in their insoluble form as a suspension to mask the taste. For example, insoluble chloramphenicol palmitate is used in the form of suspension to reduce the bitter taste of the chloramphenicol base.

Suspensions for external use are mainly lotions. This facilitates the drug application in the form of liquid which provides a fine coating of the drug to promote the action of the drug on the affected part of the skin. It is not messy to use in the form of suspensions as in the case of ointments. Calamine lotion is a good example.

Parenteral suspensions are of particular importance in the field of *depot* therapy. This is based on the slow release of the drug for extended action. This is made possible due to the size of the particle whose solubility is low and takes more time providing for sustained action. *Insulin zinc suspension* is an example.

Desirable properties of suspensions

A suspension is required to satisfy certain desirable properties so that it is acceptable. The desirable qualities are:

1. There should not be rapid settling of suspended particles
2. If the particles do settle, they must not form a hard cake at the bottom of the container and should be easily re-dispersible into uniform mixture when shaken.
3. The suspension should be easily pourable.
4. In the case of parenteral preparations, it should flow through the syringe needle
5. In the case of external preparation, it should spread easily on the surface of the skin and it must not be too fluid to run off the skin surface
6. The color and odor should be acceptable and pleasing for oral and external uses.

We are mainly concerned with the physical stability. The physical stability may be defined as the condition in which the particles do not aggregate and should remain uniformly distributed throughout the dispersion medium. Even if the particles settle, redistribution must be easy with moderate amount of agitation.

Interfacial properties

When the interfacial properties between the solid phase and the liquid phase are considered, two factors must be taken into account. They are the *surface free energy* increase resulting from increase in surface area of suspended particles due to reduction in size of particles and the *presence of electrical charges* on the surface of the dispersed solid particles in a liquid medium.

1. **Surface free energy**

The increase in surface free energy due to a reduction in size of the particles is given by the relation

$$\Delta G = \gamma \Delta A \qquad \text{... (1)}$$

where ΔG = increase in surface free energy in ergs.

ΔA = increase in surface area in cm^2

γ = interfacial tension in dynes/cm.

With excess free energy (i.e. when $\Delta G > 0$) due to increase in surface area, the system tends to approach a stable state by reducing the surface free energy spontaneously. When $\Delta G = 0$, the system is thermodynamically stable. It may be said that smaller the ΔG, the more thermodynamically stable is the suspension. A reduction in γ can be brought about by adding a wetting agent (surfactant). The molecules of the wetting agent get adsorbed between the particle and the medium and cause a reduction in interfacial tension. This produces a reduction in ΔG making the suspension stable. However, the interfacial tension cannot be made equal to zero and therefore the suspended particles in contact with liquid medium possess a finite positive interfacial tension and as a result the particles tend to flocculate or aggregate. This may be desirable or undesirable in a pharmaceutical suspension. In the event of particles remaining deflocculated, they settle relatively slowly. The settled particles tend to form eventually a hard cake at the bottom of the container. When such sediment (a hard cake like) is formed, it becomes extremely difficult to redisperse particles uniformly throughout the medium on shaking.

Be it a solid or liquid, when reduced greatly in size, there is a tendency for the particles or the globules to agglomerate or stick together. This agglomeration can occur either in air or in a liquid medium. This tendency for the agglomeration is due to excess free energy resulting out of size reduction (or comminution). When there is excess free energy, the system is thermodynamically unstable. Then, regrouping of particles to form agglomerates occurs in an attempt to reach a thermodynamically stable state. Hence, the process of agglomeration is spontaneous. In agglomerates, the particles are held together by weak *van der Waals* forces of attraction. In a liquid medium they settle and ultimately form a hard sedimented cake.

2. Electrical Properties at the surface of the dispersed particles

Both attraction and repulsion forces exist between particles dispersed in a liquid medium.

The particle-particle interaction (due to attraction and repulsion) may be given as follows.

1. The various electrostatic contributions: They may be ion-ion, ion-dipole, dipole-dipole and dipole-induced dipole. They have both attractive (between dissimilar charges) and repulsive forces (between similar charges)
2. The London dispersion forces (between atoms of one particle with those of the other. It is induced dipole-induced dipole interaction (attraction)
3. The covalent bonds (attractive)
4. *Born* repulsion forces (repulsive). It is due to overlapping of electron clouds of the atoms present in a molecule or ion.

The attractive forces due to covalent bonds and *Born repulsion forces* have an effect only when the particles are actually in touch with each other.

The London dispersion forces and hydrogen bonding forces are generally more important in describing inter-particulate behavior of non-ionic compounds in suspensions. The surface properties of the particles depend on the balance achieved between these attractive and repulsive forces.

In general, the particles in a suspension have forces of attraction which are of the London *van der Waals* type and the forces of repulsion due to the interaction of the electric double layer surrounding each particle (See under Interfacial phenomena).

The region in which the influence of the surface charge (i.e., potential) of the particle is appreciable is termed the electric double layer region. The electric double layer is considered to comprise.

1. **The Stern layer consisting of counterions:** The thickness is of the ionic dimension. The potential drop across the stern layer from the surface of the particle is sharp.
2. **The diffuse double layer:** The potential drop across this layer is somewhat gradual and it drops to zero at the end of its surface where it meets electro-neutral region.

The charged particles suspended in a liquid medium migrate towards the oppositely charged electrode under the influence of electric field. When a particle moves the counterions in the Stern layer and the solvent molecules in the solvated layer (solvent-sheath or layer called solvated layer) also move intact with the particle. That is, the plane of shear occurs at the surface of the solvated layer. This solvated layer is slightly thicker than the Stern layer.

The potential energy of the two particles (as they approach each other) may be plotted as a function of the distance of separation (Fig. 3.1). The energy of attraction (due to *London dispersion forces*) and the energy of repulsion (due to overlapping of electrical double layer) are represented in the graph as V_A and V_R respectively. The net energy (due to interaction between attractive and repulsive forces) is represented as V_n which is also the energy barrier curve. This curve has two minima and a peak. The minimum occurring at longer distance is called secondary minimum and that occurring at negligible distance is called primary minimum.

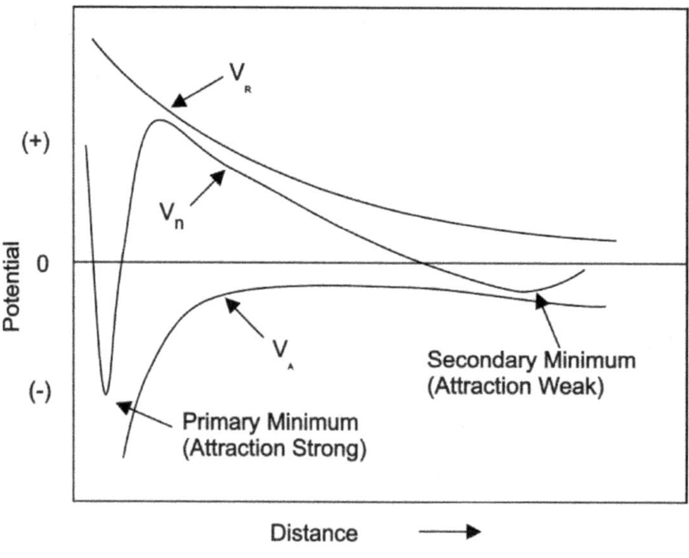

Fig. 3.1

In the presence of high repulsive energy, the potential barrier energy is also high and it prevents the collision of the approaching particles and hence, they remain deflocculated. When sedimentation of such deflocculated particles is complete, they tend to be closely packed and the particles at the bottom get compressed by the weight of the particles in the upper layer as well as by the dispersion medium. At this stage, the energy barrier is overcome and the particles come closer and closer and they enter into primary minimum. As a result, they experience attractive forces and ultimately form a hard cake like sediment. To regain the original energy barrier, a high energy is required. Hence even on vigorous agitation, the redispersion of the particles is not achieved and the particles remain as a cake.

When the particles flocculate in the secondary minimum where the attractive forces reach over the range of repulsive forces, the particles remain flocculated but are separated by a distance approximately from 1000 to 2000 Å. In the secondary minimum the particles are loosely held in floccules and are not able to enter into primary minimum since the energy barrier is too large to be surmounted.

It may be said that flocculated particles are weakly bonded and settle rapidly. The flocculated particles on sedimentation do not form a cake and are easily redispersed on shaking the container.

Flocculation and deflocculation in suspensions

The overall (or resultant) charge existing on the suspended particle is called as *zeta potential* and it is a measurable indication of the charge. Therefore, flocculation and deflocculation may be considered in terms of zeta potential. When the zeta potential is high, the particles remain dispersed and are said to be *deflocculated.* These particles resist collision due to the high zeta potential even if the particles are brought close by way of random motion or agitation.

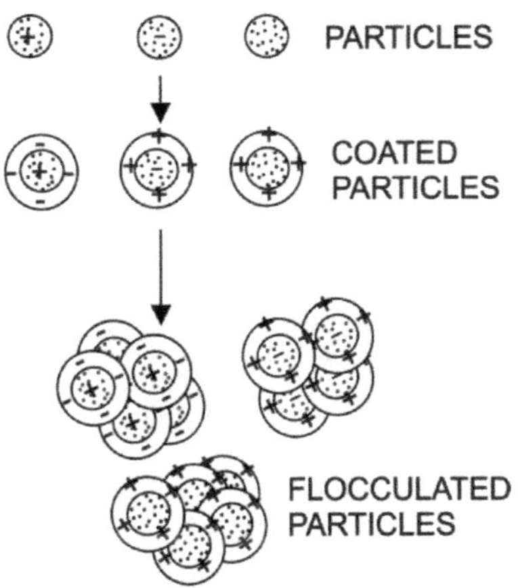

Fig. 3.2

The zeta potential can be progressively lowered by the addition of an electrolyte (whose ion which is oppositely charged to that of the suspended particles is preferentially adsorbed). At some concentration of the electrolyte, the forces of attraction dominate over the electrical forces of repulsion slightly. Under these conditions (i.e., when the zeta potential is sufficiently low), the particles form loose aggregated flocculated particles commonly called as *flocs.* (Fig.3.2) Then such a suspension is said to be *flocculated**.

(**Flocculation is a term used by some workers as aggregation in the secondary minimum and the coagulation as aggregation in the primary minimum. Zeta potential value can be determined by plotting the flocculation against the surface potential and extrapolating to zero flocculation rate.)*

The difference between *deflocculated* and *flocculated* suspensions may be given as follows (Fig. 3.3).

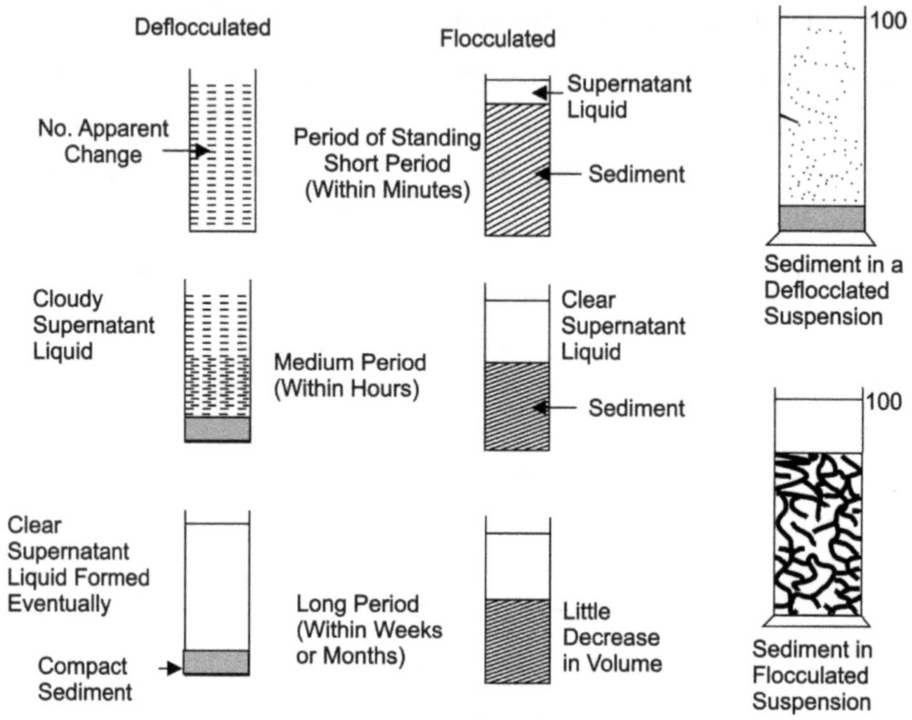

Fig. 3.3

	Deflocculated Suspension	Flocculated Suspension
1.	The particles in the suspension remain individually.	Particles form light fluffy conglomerates called flocs.
2.	Since the particles are small and remain separately, the rate of sedimentation is slow	Since the flocs are groups of particles, rate of sedimentation is fast.
3.	Formation of sediment at the bottom of the container takes a long time	Formation of sediment is quick.
4.	The sediment formed becomes eventually a hard cake	The sediment is loosely packed and presents a scaffold like structure with entrapped liquid. The sediment does not form a dense hard cake.
5.	Sediment volume is *small*	Sediment volume is *high*

6.	The supernatant liquid remains cloudy for a longer time as very small particles (approaching colloidal dimensions) take very long time to settle.	The supernatant liquid becomes clear at a shorter time since small particles are entrapped within the flocs and settle along with flocs rapidly.
7.	Redistribution of the sedimented particles by shaking the container is difficult	Redistribution of the sedimented particles by shaking the container is easy.
8.	The suspension has a pleasing appearance	The suspension is somewhat unsightly unless the sediment volume and the volume of the original suspension are equal.

Settling and its control

The sedimentation velocity of particles in a suspension is related to

1. size of the particles
2. density of the particles
3. viscosity of the dispersion medium.

The effect of these factors can be given by *Stoke's law*

$$v = \frac{d^2(\rho_s \rho_l)}{18\eta} \qquad \text{... (2)}$$

where v = average velocity of sedimentation of particles (cm/sec)

d = diameter of the particle in cm.

ρ_s *and* ρ_l = densities of the dispersed phase (solid) and the dispersion medium (liquid) respectively

g = acceleration due to gravity

η = viscosity of the dispersion medium.

Stoke's law is applicable to dilute suspensions containing spherical particles and the settling of particles should be slow with less turbulence i.e., the settling should be streamline.

Pharmaceutical suspensions being concentrated, there is disturbance for the settling of particles and hence, *Stoke's law* cannot be effectively applied. However, these factors may be expected to influence the rate of settling.

According to *Stoke's law*, settling rate for the particles may be reduced by decreasing the particle size provided the particles remain deflocculated.

The rate of sedimentation may be delayed by increasing the viscosity of the medium (by adding suitable suspending agents) as it is inversely related to the viscosity of the dispersion medium. This approach to reduce the rate of sedimentation is frequently used. However there is an optimum level for this approach as too much increase in viscosity may hinder the flow of the suspension out of the container. That is, pourability is affected and the viscosity increase may also make the redistribution of the particles uniformly throughout the dispersion medium difficult.

The other approach that may be applied is to narrow down the density difference between the dispersed particles and the dispersion medium. This is seldom possible as the density of solid particles is always greater than the liquid.

Brownian movement

When the size of the dispersed particles approaches that of colloidal dimensions, *Brownian motion* sets in. Such a *Brownian motion* may be observed if the size of the particle is reduced approximately to 2μ. However, the Brownian movement depends on the density of the particles and the density and viscosity of the dispersion medium. Considering the size of the particles normally found in most of the pharmaceutical suspensions it is unlikely that the particles will undergo *Brownian movement.*

Effect of flocculation on sedimentation rate

In a deflocculated suspension, the larger particles settle relatively at a faster rate than the smaller particles. As a result, a clear boundary is not easily discernible and the supernatant liquid remains cloudy for a considerable period of time. In the case of flocculated suspension, groups of particles are aggregated into flocs and the flocs tend to fall together while settling and there is a clear boundary formed between the sediment and the supernatant liquid. Settling in a flocculated suspension depends on size and porosity of the flocs. However, the rate of settling in a flocculated suspension is faster.

Sedimentation volume and degree of flocculation

In order to assess a formulation of suspension in terms of amount of flocculation, two parameters namely *sedimentation volume* and *degree of flocculation* are useful.

1. **Sedimentation volume**

The sedimentation volume is the ratio of ultimate volume of the sediment to the total volume of the suspension.

$$F = V_u/V_0 \quad \text{... (3)}$$

where F = sedimentation volume

V_u = ultimate volume of the sediment

V_0 = total volume of the suspension

The sedimentation volume (F) normally ranges from less than 1 to 1 and it may exceed 1. For example, if the sedimentation volume is 0.85, it means that 85% of the total volume of the suspension is occupied by the sediment (usually flocculated suspension will occupy that much of volume). When $F = 1$, the sediment volume and the total volume are equal and such a suspension is pharmaceutically acceptable. It is possible for the sedimentation volume to exceed the total volume of the suspension i.e., $F > 1$. It indicates that the network of flocs formed in the suspension is loose and fluffy that it encompasses a volume greater than the original volume of the suspension.

2. **Degree of flocculation**

Degree of flocculation is a better parameter to compare different formulations in terms of flocculation. It is the ratio of the sedimentation volume of the flocculated suspension (F) to the sedimentation volume of the suspension when deflocculated (F_α)

$$\beta = \frac{F}{F_\alpha} \quad \text{... (4)}$$

The degree of flocculation refers to the increased sediment volume because of flocculation. For example, if $\beta = 4$, the sediment volume in the flocculated suspension is increased by four times the volume of sediment in the deflocculated state. A suspension with a higher degree of flocculation is to be preferred.

Formulation of suspensions

The formulation of suspension is aimed at producing a suspension with optimal physical stability. A physically stable suspension may be produced either by

(a) the use of structured vehicle to keep the deflocculated particles in suspension, or
(b) the use of the principles of flocculation in order to assure an easy uniform redispersion of particles with minimum of agitation.

In the first approach using structured vehicles, the deflocculated particles are entrapped. This reduces the settling time and as the structured vehicle (non-Newtonian type) has shear-thinning property, redispersion is somewhat easier by shaking the container. However, when the particles ultimately settle, they form a cake at the bottom of the container making it difficult to redisperse the settled particles.

The second approach is the preparation of flocculated suspension. In this, the particles settle rapidly and the redispersion is easy. Within the time gap between the shaking of the container and the consumption, the (drug) particles may settle rapidly allowing only a dose that is subtherapeutic. As a consequence, in the formulation of suspensions, optimum physical stability may be obtained by producing suspensions with controlled flocculation in a structured vehicle.

Dispersion of particles

The first step in the formulation of suspension is the dispersion of the (drug) powder in a liquid medium. Before dispersion is undertaken, the particles should be properly wetted. Wetting is a problem with hydrophobic particles. This can be brought about by the use of wetting agents. They act by lowering the contact angle between the surface of the particle and the wetting liquid (the dispersion medium). Wetting agents are surfactants whose HLB values lie within the range of 7 to 9. The powder may be prepared as slurry in a solution of wetting agent and then the required amount of vehicle may be added to disperse the powder. Alcohol and glycerin may also be used to disperse the powder. Glycerin and similar hydrophilic substances flow into void space between the particles, coat the particles, and separate the particles bringing about dispersion. Wetting agents in smaller amounts promote wetting and deflocculation.

Controlled flocculation

The next step is to produce controlled flocculation in the suspension. Flocculation in a suspension prevents formation of a hard cake, when the particles settle down. Flocculation in a suspension may be brought about by adding

(a) electrolytes
(b) surfactants
(c) polymers

(a) **Electrolytes**: The most widely used flocculating agents are the electrolytes. When added in sufficient quantity to a well wetted and dispersed particles suspension, they (electrolytes) cause a reduction in electrical forces of repulsion bringing about flocculation in the suspension. Electrolytes reduce the electric barrier and thereby produce a reduction in zeta potential on the dispersed particles. The addition of electrolyte must be judicious so that zeta potential is reduced to a level which brings about flocculation resulting in maximum sedimentation volume.

Consider a suspension in which the particles are dispersed in an aqueous medium and the particles carry positive charges with high zeta potential (Fig. 3.4). The particles in the suspension remain deflocculated due to high zeta potential. If monobasic potassium phosphate is added to the suspension, the negatively charged phosphate ions get adsorbed on the particles bringing down the potential. This effect causes the particles to flocculate and the sediment volume is increased. On the addition of increased amounts of the electrolyte (i.e., monobasic potassium phosphate), the zeta potential gradually falls to zero and then the charge on the particle becomes negative (i.e. overall charge gets reversed). Until now, the suspension remains flocculated. But on increasing the negative charge with further addition of the electrolyte, the particles again get deflocculated since the zeta potential is increased on the negative side (Fig.3.4). The results of both the effects mentioned above are presented in Fig. 3.4 and 3.5.

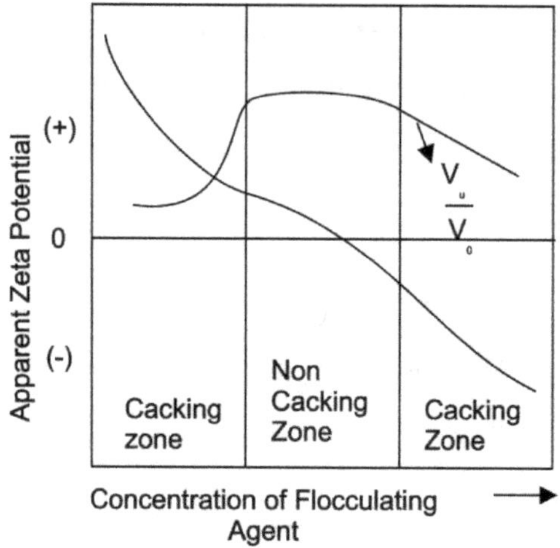

Fig. 3.4

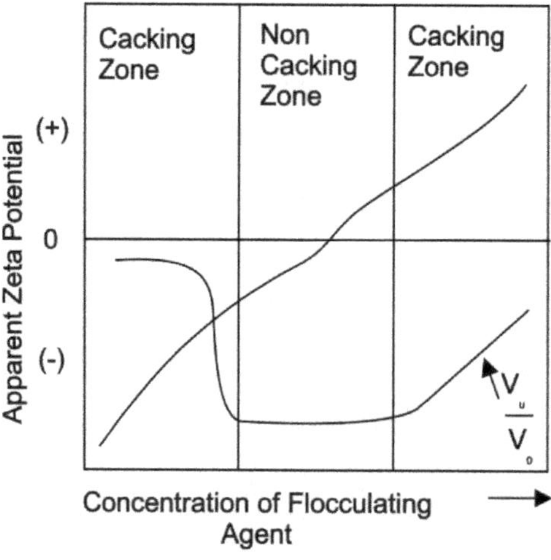

Fig. 3.5

Similarly, if the particles in a suspension are negatively charged initially, the addition of aluminium chloride brings about the effect shown (Fig. 3.5). That is the negative charge is progressively reduced by the addition of aluminium chloride as the aluminium ions (positively charged) get adsorbed on the particles. On sufficient addition of aluminium chloride, the zeta potential reaches zero and then the charge reverses and increases in the positive direction (Fig.3.4).

In both the cases, when zeta potential is high, the particles remain deflocculated and the sediment volume is less. This sediment eventually forms a hard cake making redistribution of the suspension difficult on shaking the container. On reduction in zeta potential by the addition of the electrolyte, the particles form flocs. It may be observed that the onset of flocculation is coincident with the maximum sedimentation volume. This volume virtually remains constant until the zeta potential does not exceed the critical potential value i.e., zetapotential. When it becomes sufficiently high on the opposite side, the sedimentation volume starts to fall indicating deflocculation and the sediment eventually forms a cake.

These effects have been demonstrated with bismuth subnitrate suspension (in which the particles carry positive charge initially) and sulfamerazine suspension in which the drug (sulfamerazine) particles carry negative charge initially as in the figures shown above.

(b) **Surfactants**: Flocculation have been brought about by using both ionic and non-ionic surfactants. However, the concentration of these surfactants to achieve flocculation is critical because they act as wetting agents also to bring about dispersion of the powder particles in a dispersion medium.

(c) **Polymers**: Polymers act as flocculating agents by forming a `bridge' between particles. The sedimentation volume is higher in a suspension in which polymers have been used to bring about flocculation e.g., Xanthum gum

Flocculation in structured vehicle

A suspension with controlled flocculation may look unsightly because the sediment volume will be lower than the total volume of the suspension. An ideal formulation would be a suspension with controlled flocculation supported in a structured vehicle.

To a suspension in which the particles have been flocculated to a desired degree, a polymer which is lyophilic is added to obtain a structured vehicle. Most of the pharmaceutical suspensions are prepared in aqueous medium and hence a hydrophilic polymer is used to form structured vehicle. Some examples of hydrophilic polymers are carboxy methyl cellulose, carbopol, veegum, tragacanth, bentonite etc.

The structured vehicle forming hydrophilic colloids are negatively charged and are compatible with suspensions which have been flocculated with anion of the electrolyte (For example PO_4^{-3} of monobasic potassium phosphate). That is, if the suspended particles carry a positive charge initially and are flocculated with monobasic potassium phosphate, a hydrophilic polymer may be added to form structured vehicle. Otherwise, to a suspension (with particles carrying negative charge) which has been flocculated with aluminium chloride, if a hydrophilic polymer is added, it results in an incompatible product. Under such conditions, the sign of the particle (negative charge) may be changed to positive sign and then a hydrophilic polymer may be added after flocculating the particles with the use of anion of an electrolyte. The change in sign (from negative to positive) may be brought about by using hydrophilic protective colloid. (This is similar in mechanism of protecting a hydrophobic colloid with hydrophilic colloid).

In general, a physically stable suspension may be produced

(a) by reducing the particle size by a suitable method

(b) by adding a suitable suspending agent to increase the viscosity of the medium to an optimum level and

(c) by the use of suitable quantity of proper electrolyte to cause flocculation to a desired level in a structured vehicle. The agents used to produce structured vehicle invariably may also act as suspending agents.

(d) Due to temperature fluctuations, during storage, there may be change in particle size distribution and polymorphic forms. They are the destabilizing processes. The growth in particle is termed "*Oswald ripening*" and this occurs during storage. This may alter absorption rate and in turn bioavailability of drugs. When temperature is raised, crystals of most drugs may dissolve and form supersaturated solution, which favor crystal growth. This can be prevented by adding certain polymers or surfactants. Sulphathiazole and acetaminophen crystal growth can be prevented by the addition of high molecular weight polyvinyl pyrrolidone. The molecules of the polymer attach to the free space of drug crystal lattice and form a non-condensed net like film over the drug crystal. In addition, the polymer is surrounded by a hydration shell. Thus, the crystal growth is prevented as shown in Fig. 3.6.

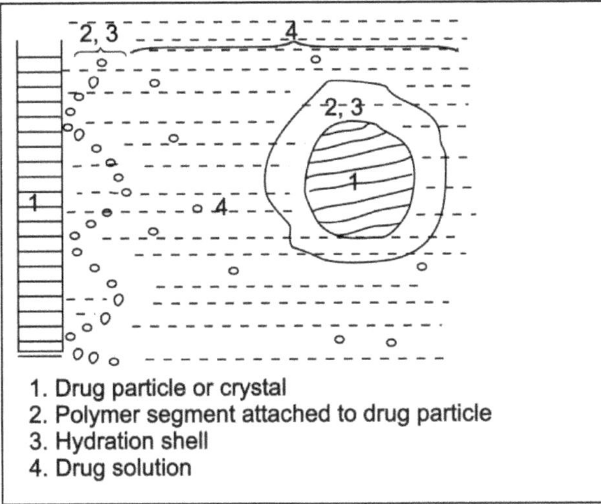

Fig. 3.6

(e) Stability of suspension may also decrease owing to interaction with excipients dissolved in the dispersion medium. **Example 1.** In sulfamerazine suspension containing non-ionic surfactant as wetting agent, sorbitol is used as flocculating agent. The amount of sorbitol required depends upon the cloud point of surfactant. The lower the cloud point, the less sorbital is needed to induce flocculation. **Example 2.** Charge on the preservative: Cetyl pyridinium chloride (a cationic surfactant) is used as preservative in suspensions. If more quantity is added, the positive charge on the preservative may reverse the charge of the dispersed particles (eg. Negatively charged zinc oxide may get reversed on the addition of cetyl pyridinium chloride). If the preservative molecules get adsorbed on the suspended particles, free fraction of preservatives in water gets reduced and this also leads to lesser preservation.

Chemical stability

In suspensions, the suspended particles are practically insoluble in the liquid vehicle and hence the chances of chemical reaction are very less. But, many drugs in suspension have a finite solubility and so may be susceptible to degradation. However, it may be assumed that the dissolution is not rate-limiting on degradation.

Thus, in order to get a stable suspension at the time of formulation as well as during storage all the above factors should be taken into account.

Rheologic properties of Suspensions

The principles of rheology are applicable to the flow properties of the suspensions. The flow property of a suspension becomes important as it is required to pour the suspension out of the container to withdraw a dose of the product. It is also important in the case of external preparations which are suspensions, as they must spread properly over the affected area when applied.

The viscosity as well as change in flow properties of the suspension will affect the rheological properties of the suspension greatly. Ideally, a suspension should have a high viscosity at low shear rates and a low viscosity at high shear rates. In a suspension under storage, the only shear is due to settling of particles. At this low shear rate, the viscosity of the suspension must be high. During shaking of the bottle, a high shear rate is produced and at this high shear rate, the viscosity should fall to a low value. Such a property may be derived from pseudo-plastic substances such as tragacanth, sodium alginate and sodium carboxy methyl cellulose which are used as suspending agents.

However, a suspending agent which is thixotropic as well as pseudoplastic may have the property of forming a gel on standing and becoming fluid when shaken. Thus a suspension containing such a combination of suspending agents may prove to be an ideal one. Such a combination of property may be obtained from a mixture of bentonite (which is thixotropic) and carboxy methyl cellulose (which is pseudoplastic).

Pharmaceutical applications of suspensions

(a) *For oral use:* A suspension provides convenient means of administering an insoluble drug as compared to tablets or capsules as far as swallowing is concerned. For adsorptive or antacid properties, usually suspensions are fast acting because of more surface area. e.g. Kaolin, magnesium carbonate, calcium carbonate and magnesium trisilicate. Insoluble derivatives of drugs are often used to reduce the unpleasant taste. e.g., Chloramphenicol palmitate. Insoluble drugs which are susceptible to hydrolysis are dispensed as dry syrups and are reconstituted with water at the time of use. e.g., *Ampicillin dry syrup*.

(b) *For external use:* Number of lotions are of suspension type (e.g., calamine lotion for protective action on the skin). Semisolid suspensions are pastes (e.g., Magnesium sulfate paste, Zinc and salicyclic acid paste, Tooth paste etc). The performance and acceptability of these preparations depend upon the sedimentation and rheological properties.

(c) *For injections:* Insoluble drugs which are susceptible to hydrolysis are dispersed as sterile powders in vials. At the time of their use, they are reconstituted with sterile water for injection. e.g., *Penicillin injection.* Suspension injections provide for sustained action. e.g., *Streptomycin oily injections.*

2. EMULSIONS

An emulsion is a dispersion of a liquid as globules in another liquid, both the liquids being immiscible with each other. (Example: dispersion of oil in water or dispersion of water in oil). The diameters of the globules usually vary from 0.1 to 10 μm, although globule diameters as small as 0.01 μm and as large as 100 μm are possible in some emulsions. Emulsions having globules of mean diameter about 5 μm are called fine emulsions and emulsions with large globules are referred to as coarse emulsions. The emulsion is said to be thermodynamically unstable since the globules coalesce and the phases will ultimately separate. To stabilize an emulsion, a third substance called emulgent or emulsifier or emulsifying agent is invariably added to the emulsion. Therefore, *an emulsion may be defined as a biphasic system consisting of two immiscible liquids of which one is dispersed as fine globules throughout the other with the help of suitable emulsifying agent or agents.* The emulsion may be a dilute dispersion, a concentrated dispersion or semisolid. The liquid emulsions are opaque, milky white, and viscous. The particle diameter of the disperse phase are usually from about 0.1μ to 10 μm, although the particle diameters as small as 0.01μm and as large as 100 μm are found. The semisolid emulsions are called creams.

Types of emulsion

In an emulsion one liquid phase is essentially polar (aqueous) while the other liquid is relatively non polar (e.g., oil).

(a) Oil in Water emulsion

(a) When the oil is distributed as globules throughout the aqueous continuous phase, the emulsion is called oil in water (o/w) type emulsions. (Fig.3.7) Medicinal emulsions for oral administrations are usually o/w type emulsions. Emulsions are preferred to mask the unpleasant odour and taste of certain medicinal oils and also to increase the absorption. Absorption of shark liver oil is facilitated when given in the form of emulsion. The various emulsifying agents used for producing o/w type emulsions are acacia gum (has more of emulsifying property and less of viscosity building property and hence called primary emulsifying agent), tragacanth gum (has more of viscosity building property and less of emulsifying property and hence called secondary emulsifying agent), starch, methyl cellulose, sodium carboxy methyl cellulose, soluble salts of alginic acid and gelatin. Finely divided solid such as aluminium hydroxide yields o/w type emulsions (*Liquid Paraffin Magnesium Hydroxide Emulsion*). Non-ionic surfactants such as tweens and natural emulsifying agents such as acacia, sodium carboxy methyl cellulose are used in oral emulsions.

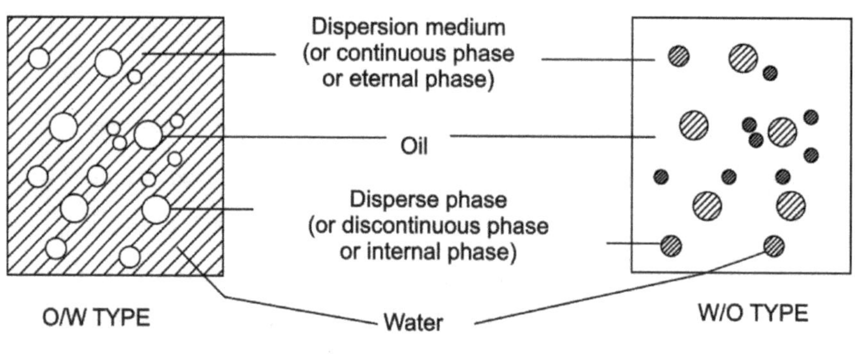

Fig. 3.7

O/w type emulsions may also be used externally Ex. *Turpentine Liniment and Vanishing Cream*. The various emulsifying agents are sodium lauryl sulfate, triethanolamine stearate, monovalent soaps like sodium oleate, glyceryl monostearete mixed with a monovalent soap or alkyl sulfate etc. Surfactants or mixture of surfactants having HLB values in the range 8-16 will yield o/w type emulsions.

(b) Water-in-oil emulsion

When water is distributed as globule in oily continuous phase, the emulsion is called water in oil type emulsion (w/o emulsion) (Fig. 3.7). These emulsions are mainly for external use. Certain food such as butter and some salad dressings are w/o emulsions. The w/o emulsions used externally are Cold cream, Oily Calamine Lotion, Oily Zinc Cream etc. The various emulsifying agents used are polyvalent soaps like calcium palmitate, sorbitan esters (spans), cholesterol and wool fat. A surfactant (or a mixture of surfactants), whose HLB value is between 3 and 6 yields w/o type emulsions.

(c) Multiple emulsion or complex emulsions

In this oil globules surrounded by water layer are dispersed as complex globules in continuous oil medium (i.e., o/w/o) or water globules surrounded by oil layer are dispersed as complex globules in continuous water medium (w/o/w). It is only of theoretical importance. In multiple emulsions both hydrophobic and hydrophilic emulsifiers are used. O/W/O emulsions are formed better by lipophilic non-ionic surfactant using gum acacia emulsified systems.

W/O/W emulsions may be prepared first by forming W/O emulsion from isopropyl myristate (oil), sorbitan-mono-oleate (emulgent) and distilled water. Then, the emulsion is added to a polyoxyethelene sorbitan mono oleate solution in water to produce finally W/O/W emulsion - a multiple emulsion. Such multiple emulsions may be used for prolonged action, taste masking, more effective dosage forms, parenteral preparations, protection of the drug against external environment and enzyme entrapment.

(d) Micro emulsions

These emulsions are clear transparent solutions. They appear to represent a state intermediate between thermodynamically stable solubilized solutions and thermodynamically unstable emulsions. They contain droplets of oil in water phase (o/w) or droplets of water in oil phase (w/o) with diameters of about 10 to 200 nm and the volume fraction of the dispersed phase varies from 0.2 to 0.8.

For making micro emulsion with a surfactant, a co-surfactant is also used. An anionic surfactant (sodium lauryl sulfate or potassium oleate) is dispersed in an organic liquid such as benzene and a small amount of water is added. The gradual addition of pentanol (lipophilic co-surfactant) to the above gives a clear solution at 30°C. The surfactants form an adsorbed film on the microemulsion particles to prevent coalescence. Thus, the micro emulsion contains a large or swollen micelles containing the internal phase similar to solubilized solutions. The globule size of the internal phase may also be reduced by using sonication or ultra-frequency waves. Usually the emulgent should be 20 to 30% of the weight of the oil used. In the preparation of W/O systems, oil is blended with the emulgent and the water is added to produce the emulsion. Micro emulsions are used for solubilization of drugs in pharmaceutical systems, for making some cosmetics, also used in food industries, and for making wax polishing products.

Recently micro-emulsions are being studied as drug delivery systems. They may be used to increase bioavailability of drugs poorly soluble in water by incorporation of the drug in the internal phase. Micro emulsions have also been considered as topical drug delivery system and the experiments revealed that delivery of certain drugs from microemulsions was faster and showed deeper penetration into the skin. Several patents were made by scientists for topical delivery of certain antihypertensive and anti-inflammatory drugs formulated in microemulsions.

Applications of emulsions

1. Medicinal agents which have objectionable taste and odour (for example, shark liver oil, castor oil, olive oil etc.) may be formulated into o/w emulsions to mask the taste and to make palatable.
2. Oil soluble vitamins (A, D, E and K) are absorbed more completely when they are made into fine emulsions than when they are administered as oily solutions.
3. O/w type emulsions are used as a dosage form for intravenous administration of oils and fats with high calorific value to patients who cannot ingest food by other means and the globules in this emulsion should be similar to the size of chylomicrons (nearly colloidal size). The choice of emulsifying agent for intravenous emulsions are restricted. The emulgents used may be gelatin, lecithins and some non-ionic surfactants. Only edible oils are used as oily phases.
4. Radio-opaque emulsions are being used as diagnostic agents in X-ray examination.
5. Emulsions of both the types (o/w and w/o) are extensively used to prepare pharmaceutical preparation for external use and as cosmetic preparations. Such a product should be easily spreadable, water washable non-staining and more acceptable to the patients. E.g., Cold cream and vanishing cream.

6. Emulsification is used in aerosol products to produce foams. The propellant that forms the dispersed liquid phase within the container vaporizes when the emulsion is discharged from the container.
7. Emulsions afford protection to drugs susceptible to oxidation or hydrolysis.
8. Liquid paraffin is used as purgative when taken orally and is not absorbed. It should not be made into fine emulsion since fine globules may be absorbed.
9. Some enemas are made as emulsions either for local action (E.g., soap enemas) or to influence drug action.
10. Solid drugs which show poor solubility may be dissolved in the oil and emulsified. From this emulsion, the bioavailability is more (as compared to tablet or suspension. E.g., non-steroidal antifungal agents).

Identification of type of emulsions

Mainly the emulsions are either o/w type or w/o type. They may be identified by the following tests.

(a) Dilution test

Generally, addition of the continuous phase to an emulsion will lead to dilution and the addition of internal phase to an emulsion will lead to separation of the added liquid.

Accordingly, addition of water to o/w type emulsion leads to dilution of emulsion without any separation of added water. However, separation will occur with w/o type emulsion. Similarly, addition of oil to o/w type emulsion leads to separation of the added oil. However, dilution occurs with w/o type emulsion by the addition of oil.

(b) Dye test

A small quantity of water-soluble dye such as methylene blue or brilliant blue may be dusted on the surface of an emulsion. If the emulsion is of o/w type the dye will dissolve in the continuous phase and diffuse throughout the water. If the emulsion is of w/o type, the water-soluble dye will lie in clumps on the surface.

Alternatively, a small quantity of oil soluble dye may be added to the emulsion and shaken. If a drop of the emulsion is examined under microscope, the external phase is stained indicating the emulsion is w/o. If the internal phase is stained (i.e., colored spots may be seen), the emulsion is o/w type.

In a similar manner, the test can be carried out with water soluble dye.

(c) *Electrical conductivity test*

Water is a good conductor of electricity especially when it contains dissolved electrolytes whereas oil is a bad conductor of electricity. This fact is utilized to find out the type of emulsion.

An electrical circuit is shown in the Fig: 3.8. The emulsion is kept in a vessel with two electrodes dipped in. It is connected to a battery, switch and a bulb in series. The circuit is closed by switching on. If the bulb glows continuously, it indicates that the continuous phase in the emulsion is water and the emulsion is o/w type. If the bulb flickers (not glowing continuously) the emulsion is w/o type.

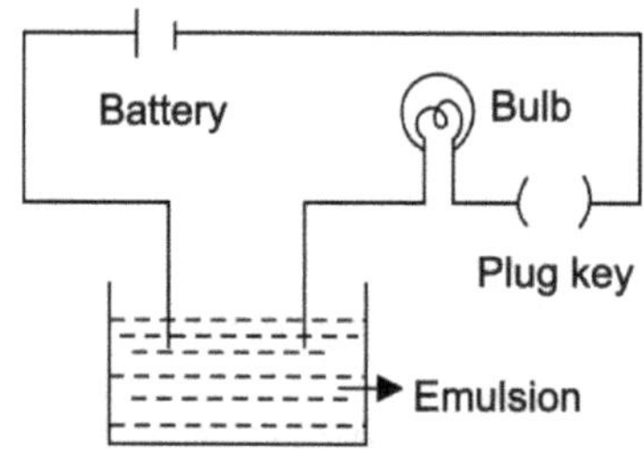

Fig. 3.8 Electrical conductivity test

(d) *By observing the creaming or sedimentation pattern in emulsion*

Creaming is the upward movement of the internal phase in an emulsion (i.e. positive creaming). Creaming occurs only in o/w emulsions. It is nothing but the separation of lower and higher density liquids. The liquid with lower density tends to move upwards. Sedimentation (negative creaming) is the downward movement of globules of the internal phase towards the bottom of the container. It occurs only in w/o type emulsion. It is also a process of separation of liquids with different densities. In this case the liquid globules with higher density (i.e water) settle at the bottom.

Theories of emulsification

There is no universal theory of emulsification. Any theory, to be meaningful, should be capable of explaining

(a) type of emulsion formed
(b) stability of emulsion

Modern approach:

The modern approach for the theory of emulsification is as follows.

When a liquid is shaken with another immiscible liquid, the liquid in small quantity disperses as fine droplets in another liquid which is in large quantity. Depending upon the agitation or the shear rate used, the size of the droplets may vary. The higher shear rates produce smaller droplets. The time of agitation is also important. The mean size of the droplets decreases rapidly in the first few seconds. The limiting size range is generally reached within one to five minutes. Such dispersion is thermodynamically instable and the two liquids separate rapidly into two clearly defined layers. It is due to the fact that the cohesive forces between the molecules of the same liquid are greater than adhesive forces between the molecules of the two different liquids. The existence of an emulsion is the result of the two competing processes - one is the dispersion of one liquid in the form of droplets throughout the other and the other is the combination of these droplets to reform initial bulk liquid. The first process increases the free energy and the second process decreases the free energy i.e. the second process is spontaneous. Therefore, for a stable emulsion, it is necessary to promote dispersion by using a well operating machinery to produce fine droplets in a short period of time and to minimize the second process by using certain parameters discussed below to stabilize emulsion.

When a liquid is broken into small particles, the interfacial area of the globules is enormous as compared to surface area of the original liquid. For example, if 1 cm^3 of mineral oil is dispersed into globules of a volume of 0.01μ (10^{-6} cm) into 1 cm^3 of water, the surface area of the oil droplets becomes 600 sq. meters. The surface free energy associated with this area is about 34×10^7 erg or 8 calories, though the total volume of the system ($2cm^2$) remains the same. Thus, the system becomes thermodynamically instable. Hence, the droplets or globules tend to flocculate (aggregation of droplets) and subsequently coalesce (fusing of the agglomerate into a larger drop). To prevent this, emulsifying agents are added to give stable coherent interfacial film surrounding each droplet and thus, stabilizes the emulsion. The emulsifying agents may be divided into three groups.

(a) ***Surface active agents.*** These are adsorbed at oil/water interface to form monomolecular films and thus reduce surface tension.

(b) ***Hydrophilic colloids.*** These are adsorbed at oil-water interface to form multimolecular film.

(c) ***Finely divided solids.*** These are adsorbed at the oil-water interface to form particulate layer.

(a) Monomolecular adsorption

Surface active agents or amphiphiles reduce interfacial tension because of their adsorption at the oil-water interface to form monomolecular layer. A good emulsifying agent will reduce the interfacial tension to 1 dyne/cm and thus the surface free energy of the system is reduced to one sixtieth of that calculated earlier. In addition to this the monomolecular layer prevent coalescence between droplets. Such a film should be flexible so that it is capable of reforming rapidly if broken. An additional effect promoting stability is the presence of a surface charge which will cause repulsion between adjacent particles.

The presence of charges on the surface of oil globules creates an electrical double layer around each globule. (Fig: 3.9) Overlapping of electrical double layer gives rise to a repulsion which opposes the *van der Waals* forces of attraction. The variation in net potential of interaction due to combined effects of repulsive and attractive forces between oil globules in an o/w emulsion is given as follows.

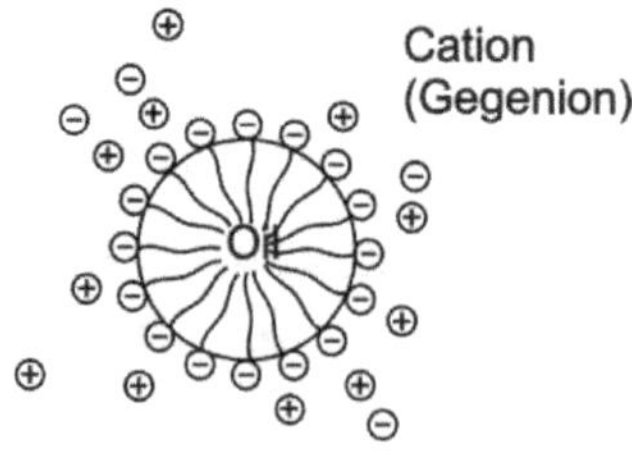

Fig. 3.9

If the potential barrier is high, globules will bounce apart. If the approaching globules are able to overcome the energy of barrier (due to thermal effects, decomposition of surfactant, addition of oppositely charged electrolytes or surfactants) they pass into primary minimum and the emulsion may break which now depends upon the strength of the adsorbed film. Flocculation may occur in the secondary minimum but the globules are separated by a layer of continuous phase. Refer Fig. 3.10

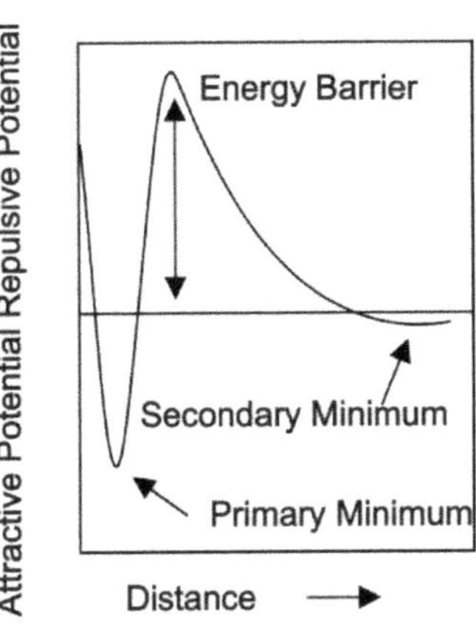

Fig. 3.10

Between the surfactant molecules adsorbed at the interface, repulsion may occur due to like charges. Hence to promote adsorption, lipophilic hydrocarbon chain of sufficient length must be present. That is why potassium stearate ($C_{17}H_{35}COOK$) has more emulsion stabilizing ability than potassium laurate ($C_{11}H_{23}COOK$). Combination of emulsifiers is preferred to a single emulsifier to produce stable emulsions.

The adsorption of a water-soluble surfactant at oil-water interface is also promoted by the presence of an oil soluble surfactant in the oily phase. The effect is mutual which leads to the formation of a closely packed film (Refer Fig.3.11) called complex condensed film which provides for more stability.

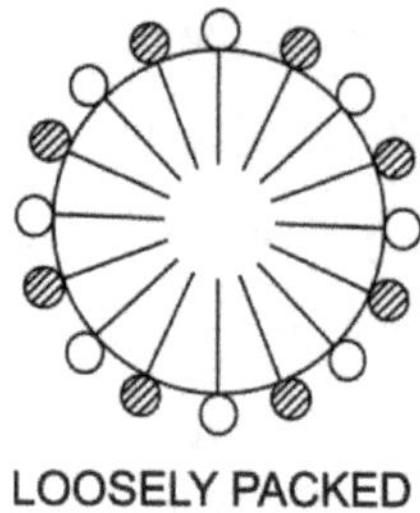

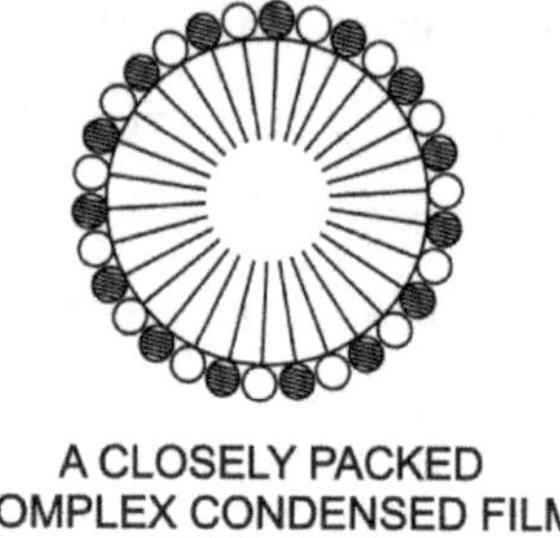

Fig. 3.11

Example:

(a) a combination of water soluble sodium lauryl sulphate (1 part) and oil soluble cetostearyl alcohol (9 parts). (It is called emulsifying wax.)

(b) a combination of water soluble cetrimide (1 part) and oil soluble cetostearyl alcohol (9 parts) (It is called cetrimide emulsifying wax)

The type of emulsion that is produced (o/w or w/o) depends upon the property of emulsifying agent. It is referred to as hydrophile lipophile balance (HLB) that is the balance between the polar and non-polar nature of the emulsifier. The HLB values of surfactants have been discussed under Interfacial phenomena.

O/w emulsion is formed when the HLB value of the emulsifier is in the range of about 8 to 16 and w/o emulsions are formed when the range is 3 to 6. For example, span 60 having a HLB value of 4.7 will produce w/o emulsion and a blend of tween 20 and span 20 having a HLB value of 12 will yield o/w emulsion. Thus, the type of emulsion is a function of relative solubility of the surface-active agent, the phase in which it is more soluble being the continuous phase. (It is called Bancroft rule). An emulsifying agent with high HLB value is soluble in water and it produces o/w emulsion and that with low HLB value is oil soluble producing w/o emulsion.

Davies has proposed that the type of emulsion formed depends on the coalescence kinetics of the two liquid phases when they are shaken together in the presence of an emulsifying agent. Say the coalescence rate of oil globules dispersed in water is rate 1 and the coalescence rate of water globules dispersed in oil is rate 2. When an emulsifying agent having a HLB value greater than 8 is used, rate 1 will be less than rate 2 and therefore, an o/w emulsion will result.

(b) *Multi molecular adsorption*

Hydrocolloids form multimolecular layer at the interface. They are strong and resist coalescence. They do not cause appreciable lowering of interfacial tension. An auxiliary effect with these hydrocolloids is the significant increase in the viscosity of the medium. Since they are hydrophilic, they promote only o/w type emulsions. Their use is limited because of availability of large number of synthetic surfactants. The mechanical strength of gel barrier may be increased by increasing gelation which is more effective at iso-electric point. With anionic hydrocolloids such as carboxy methyl cellulose, gelation is induced at low pH and the film formed is rigid.

(c) *Solid particles adsorption*

Finely divided solid particles that are wetted to some degree by both oil and water can act as emulsifying agents. They concentrate at the interface and produce a film around each droplet (particulate layer) and this effect prevents coalescence strongly because of the mechanical strength of the film. Those powders that are wetted preferentially by water form o/w emulsions and those that are wetted easily by oil tend to form w/o emulsion. An extremely rigid interfacial film of close packed particles can be produced by capillary force as shown in the diagram (Fig. 3.12).

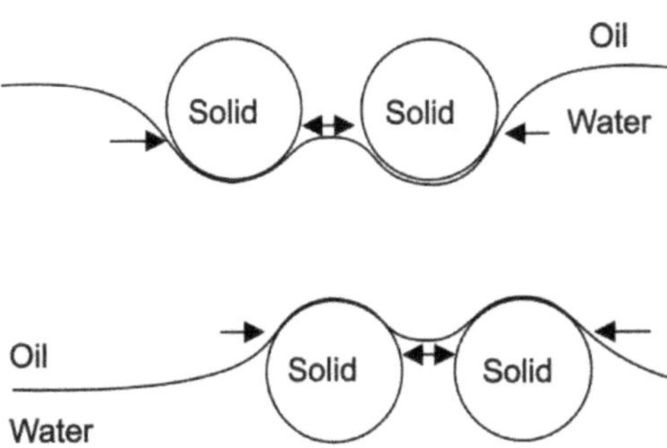

Fig. 3.12 Capillary forces cause similar particles cohere strongly

Other factors influencing stability of emulsions

Electrical double layer: In the case of w/o emulsion, ionization of substances in oil is weak. However ***electrical double layer*** may be formed in the water globules dispersed in the oil.

The diffuse part of such layers is thick. Hence, potential energy barrier to flocculation is lower in w/o than in o/w emulsions. Flocculation occurs more easily in w/o type emulsion.

Solvation effects: The hydrophilic groups of adsorbed emulsifier may have thick solvation sheaths which aid in the prevention of flocculation of oil globules. Another school of thought is that solvation sheath of short range do not contribute to stability of emulsion.

Stearic effects: Hydrophilic group of many non-ionic emulsifying agents consists of extensive poly ethylene oxide chains. Oil globules carrying adsorbed molecules of this type behave in a manner that they are coated with a thick layer of hydrophilic colloid which prevents flocculation of oil globules.

Emulsifying agents

One of the important components in emulsion is the emulsifying agent. An emulsifying agent should have the following desirable properties.

(a) Should have effective surface-active property and should reduce surface tension to below 10 dyne/cm.

(b) Should get adsorbed quickly around the droplets (or globules) as a condensed, non-adherent film which will prevent coalescence.

(c) Should impart the droplet an adequate electric potential so that mutual repulsion results

(d) Should increase the viscosity of the emulsion

(e) Should be effective in a reasonably low concentration

(f) Should be non-toxic

(g) Should be odorless and tasteless and if there is taste and odour, they should be compatible with the product.

(h) Should have good chemical stability

(i) Should be compatible with the other ingredients in the emulsion.

Type	Type of film	Examples
Synthetic surfactants	Monomolecular	**1. Anionic** *Soaps:* Potassium laureate and triethanolamine stearate. *Sulphates:* Sodium lauryl sulphate and alkyl poly oxyethylene sulphate

		Sulfonates: Dioctyle sodium sulphosuccinate **2. Cationic:** Quaternary ammonium compounds Cetyltrimethyl ammonium bromide **3. Nonionic** polyoxyethylene dathy alcohol ethers sorbitan fatty esters poly oxyethylene sorbitan fatty acid esters.
Natural	Multimolecular	**Hydrophilic colloids:** Acacia, gelatin
	Monomolecular	Cholesterol, Lecithin
Finely divided solids	Solid particle (particulate layer)	**Colloidal clays:** Bentonite, veegum, Metallic hydroxides magnesium hydroxide.

Auxiliary emulsifying agents

Name	Composition	Uses
Bentonite	Colloidal hydrated aluminium silicate	Hydrophilic thickening agents and stabiliser for o/w and w/o lotions and creams.
Cetyl alcohol	Chiefly $C_{16}H_{33}OH$	Lipophilic thickening agent and stabiliser for o/w lotions and liniments.
Glyceryl mono stearate	$C_{17}H_{35}COOCH_2$ CHOH CH2OH	
Magnesium hydroxide	$Mg(OH)_2$	Hydrophilic stabiliser for o/w emulsions.
Methyl cellulose	Series of methyl esters of cellulose	Hydrophilic thickening agent and stabiliser for o/w emulsions. It is a weak o/w emulsifier.
Silice gel	Hydrous oxides of silica	Hydrophilic stabiliser in ointments

Sodium alginate	Sodium salt of alginic acid, a purified carbohydrate extracted from giant kelp.	Hydrophilic thickening agent and stabiliser for o/w emulsion.
Sodium carboxy methyl cellulose	Sodium salt of carboxy methyl esters of cellulose	"
Stearic acid	A mixture of solid acids and fats, chiefly stearic and palmitic	
Stearyl alcohol	Chiefly $C_{18}H_{37}OH$	Lipophilic thickening agent and stabiliser for o/w lotions and ointments.
Tragacanth	Dried gummy exudate of the species Astragalus	Hydrophilic thickening agent and stabiliser for o/w emulsions. It is a weak o/w emulsifier.
Veegum	Colloidal magnesium aluminium silicate	Hydrophilic thickening agent and stabiliser for o/w lotion and creams.

Calculation of the amount of the emulsifier for an emulsion

The concentration of the emulsifier required to form a condensed film around the droplets of the dispersed phase to give a stable emulsion is calculated as follows.

Say 100 gm of an oil having a density of 1 is to be emulsified in 100 ml of water.

If the desired particle diameter (i.e. of droplet diameter) is 1μ, then the particle diameter in terns of cm is 1×10^{-4} cm.

Volume of particle

$$= \frac{\pi d^3}{6} = 0.524 \times 10^{-12} \text{cm}^3$$

Total number of particles in 100 grams.

$$= \frac{100}{0.524 \times 10^{-12}}$$

$$= 191.0 \times 10^{12}$$

Surface area of each particle = πd^2

$$= 3.142 \times (1 \times 10^{-4})^2 \text{cm}^2$$

$$= 3.142 \times 10^{-8} \text{ cm}^2$$

Total surface area

$$= 3.142 \times 10^{-8} \times 191.0 \times 10^{12}$$

$$= 600 \times 10^{4} \text{ cm}^2$$

If the area that each molecule occupies at the oil-water interface is 30×10^{-16}cm^2

we require $\frac{600 \times 10^4}{30 \times 10^{-16}} = 2 \times 10^{21}$ molecules.

Suppose the molecular weight of the emulsifying agent is 1000, then the required weight is

$$\frac{1000 \times 2 \times 10^{21}}{6.023 \times 10^{23}} = 3.32 \text{ grams.}$$

This calculation may serve as a guide to determine the weight of emulsifying agent (approximately) needed for the preparation of an emulsion.

Selection of emulsifying agent for various uses

Selection of an emulsifying agent depends on the use to which the emulsion is required. For example, emulsifying agent may be required for an emulsion meant for internal, external or parenteral use. Medicinal emulsions for internal use usually of the o/w type. The emulsifying agents are mostly synthetic nonionic surfactants, and natural surfactants such as acacia, tragacanth, and gelatin. Emulsions meant for external use may be o/w or w/o types. The o/w type emulsion for external use may contain synthetic nonionic surfactants, sodium lauryl sulfate, tri-ethanolamine stearate, monovalent soaps such as sodium glyceryl monostrearate mixed with a small amount of an alkylsulfate. Pharmaceutical w/o emulsions are used almost exclusively for external application and may contain polyvalent soaps such as calcium palmitate, sorbitan esters (spans), cholesterol, and wool fat as emulsifiers. For parenteral use the emulsifier, lecithin (which is a mixture of phospholipids having a negative charge at physiologic pH) is used,

Formulation of emulsion by HLB method

The factors to be considered in the formulation of emulsion may be

1. The type of emulsion with respect the nature of the drug and use
2. The emulsifying agent or agents

3. Other components needed for formulation
4. Compatibility between the components of the emulsion

Taking it for granted that the other factors have been satisfied for the formulation of emulsion, we shall concentrate on the selection of the emulsifying agent or agents, because it of prime importance in the successful formulation of an emulsion.

The type of emulsion o/w or w/o that is produced, depends primarily on the property of the emulsifying agent or agents. The characteristic property is referred to as ***hydrophilic – lipophilic balance*** (HLB). The HLB portrays the polar – non-polar nature of the emulsifier.

When the disperse phase is broken into smaller globules or droplets, the interfacial area of the globules in contact with the dispersion or external phase constitute a surface area that is enormous compared with the original surface area (of the disperse or internal phase) before globules formation. (*for example, if* $1cm^3$ *or 1ml of an oil is mixed with* $1cm^3$ *or 1ml of water to produce small globules of* $0.01\mu m$*, the total surface area of the globules will be about* $600m^2$). The increase in surface area increases the surface free energy and the system becomes thermodynamically unstable. As a result, the globules or droplets have a tendency to coalesce. To prevent this coalescence, it is necessary to introduce an emulsifying agent or agents. On introduction of the emulsifier or emulsifiers, the molecules of the emulsifier or emulsifiers move of their own accord to the interface and surround the oil globules (i.e. get adsorbed on to the surface of the oil globules) bringing down the interfacial tension. In order to accomplish, the emulsifier or emulsifiers should have the required HLB (i.e., RHLB) value.

Griffin has provided a logical means of selecting emulsifiers. This method, based on the balance between hydrophilic and lipophilic portions of the emulsifiers, is now widely used and has come to be known as the HLB system. It is mostly used in the rational selection of combination of non-ionic emulsifiers.

1. For o/w emulsion, emulsifier or combination of emulsifiers with an HLB range of 8 to 18 may be selected.

2. For w/o emulsion, emulsifier or combination of emulsifiers with an HLB range of 4 to 8 may be selected.

Griffin has also evolved a series of required HLB values for oils and the related materials to be emulsified with emulsifier or emulsifiers. If the HLB of oil (internal phase) is 10.5, then an emulsifier with HLB value of 10.5 can be selected. If a mixture of emulsifiers, say two, is intended to produce the HLB value of 10.5, an emulsifier A with a low HLB value (say 4.3) and an emulsifier B with a high HLB value (say15.0) are selected. Then, a blend of these two emulsifiers can be found by alligation method shown below.

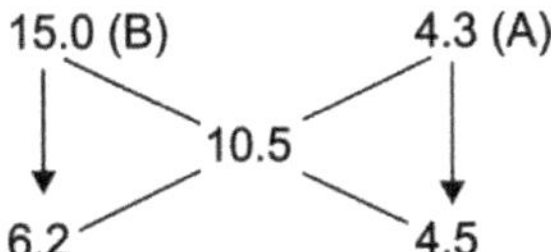

A mixture of 4.5 parts by weight of the emulsifier A and 6.2 parts by weight of emulsifier B will give the required HLB value of 10.5. When carrying out preliminary investigation with a particular material (i.e., oil) to be emulsified, it is better to try several pairs of emulsifiers to obtain the best formulation.

If the HLB value of the oil (internal or disperse phase) is not known, various blends of the emulsifying agents are prepared to obtain a wide range of HLB mixture with different HLB values. The HLB blend that gives the best emulsion on the basis of physical stability is taken as the HLB value of the oil. This procedure may be repeated with the combinations of another pair of emulsifiers to confirm the value of HLB for the oil. The difference should be within ± 1 unit. Thus, finding the required HLB value for the oil, the emulsion can be prepared.

The HLB system, however, gives no information as to the amount of emulsifier required. Having once determined the correct blend of emulsifying agents required to emulsify the internal phase, another series of emulsions, all at the same HLB, but with increasing concentrations of the emulsifier blends are prepared. The minimum concentration that gives the required degree of physical stability is selected.

Stability of emulsions

Stability of emulsions is characterized by

(a) absence of coalescence of internal phase
(b) absence of creaming
(c) maintenance of elegance with respect to color, odor and other physical properties.

The various instabilities of the emulsions are

(A) flocculation and creaming
(B) coalescence and breaking
(C) phase inversion.

(A) Flocculation and Creaming

Creaming results from flocculation and concentration of globules of the internal phase. If the disperse phase is less dense than the continuous phase (o/w type emulsion) a creamy layer (containing concentrated globules of the internal phase) collects at the top of the emulsion since the velocity of sedimentation becomes negative. It is called upward creaming. In the case of w/o type emulsion, creaming occurs in a downward direction since the velocity of sedimentation is positive i.e. sedimentation of the dispersed globules takes place. Creaming occurs as a result of density difference between the dispersed phase and the dispersion medium. Creaming is not a serious problem since it is reversible and redistribution (or redispersion) of the internal phase occurs on shaking the container.

The rate of sedimentation of a droplet particle is governed by ***Stoke's law***. According to this law, the rate of creaming may be decreased by increasing the viscosity of the dispersion medium using viscosity improvers or thickening agent such as methyl cellulose, tragacanth, and sodium alginate. The particle size of the globules may be reduced by homogenization. If the average particle size of the emulsion is reduced, the rate of creaming is reduced considerably. If the globules are reduced to a diameter below 2 to 5 μ, Brownian movements may set in. Adjusting the density difference between two phases (i.e. oil and water) also increases the stability but this method is not suitable for pharmaceutical preparations. Creaming of emulsion is also called sedimentation pattern of emulsions.

(B) Coalescence and breaking

The coalescence (aggregation of globules into larger drops) of the dispersed particles lead to complete separation of oil and water. It is a serious problem since redistribution does not take place on shaking the container.

Factors causing breaking

(a) A substance which is incompatible with the emulsifier, destroys the emulsifier ability. Example: effect of large anions on cationic emulsifier, effect of calcium and magnesium ions on monovalent soaps, effect of phenolic substances on ceto-macrogol.

(b) On increasing the temperature, the number of collisions between globules will increase leading to cracking or breaking of the emulsion. This is because the energy barrier between the globules is overcome by thermal effects. It is made use of in accelerated stability tests on the stability of emulsion.

(c) Increased temperature may coagulate certain type of macro molecular emulsifying agents.

(d) Freezing of aqueous phase will produce ice crystals which exert pressure on globules.

(e) Attempt to incorporate excessive amounts of disperse phase may cause breaking of emulsion causing the globules to coalesce.

(C) Phase volume ratio

It has a secondary influence on the stability of the emulsion. It refers to the relative volumes of internal and external phases in the emulsion. The volume of uniform sized globules of the internal phase in its closest packing cannot theoretically exceed 74% of the total volume of the emulsion. This value is known as *critical value*. It is defined as the volume of the internal phase above which the emulsifying agent cannot produce a stable emulsion. In some emulsions, the value may be higher than 74% because of irregular shape and size of the globules. Generally, a phase volume ratio of 50/50 (or 50:50) results in about the most stable emulsion. Attempts to incorporate more than about 74% of oil in o/w emulsion will lead to cracking.

A o/w emulsion stabilized with sodium stearate can be inverted to w/o type by adding calcium chloride to form calcium stearate. Inversion of o/w emulsion into w/o type emulsion and *vice versa* is called *inversion of emulsion*

Inversion may also be produced by alterations in phase volume ratio. For example, an o/w emulsifier is mixed with oil and a little quantity of water, a w/o type emulsion is produced by agitation. Since water volume is less, it forms w/o emulsion. But when more water is added slowly, phase inversion occurs and o/w type emulsion is produced. Inversion has also been observed when an emulsion which has been prepared by heating and mixing the two phases, is cooled. It is due to the temperature dependent changes in the solubilities of the emulsifying agents. Phase inversion can be prevented by choosing proper emulsifying agent in suitable concentration. Wherever possible, it is better to see the internal phase does not exceed 50% of total volume of the emulsion.

Phase inversion technique is sometimes used to produce emulsions with fine droplet sizes.

In short, the most important factor in the stabilization of emulsions is the reduction in interfacial tension to a large extent possible. This can be achieved with an emulsifying agent, which forms a tough and elastic film around the globules of the internal phase. A suitable combination of emulsifying agents can also be used

Preservation of emulsions

Antimicrobial agents are added for preservation of emulsions to protect against microbial attack. Frequently, a preservative exhibits a lower antimicrobial activity in an emulsion than in a solution. It is because of the `partitioning effect' of the agent between the oil and water. This effect causes a lowering of the effective concentration of the antimicrobial agent in water. Hence sufficient additional amount of antimicrobial agent should be added to make amends for the amount partitioned into the oily phase so as to get the `effective concentration' of the antimicrobial agent in the aqueous phase. The chemical stability of the various components of emulsion is also important since some materials may be more prone to degradation in the emulsified state than they are in the bulk solution.

Rheological properties of emulsions

Rheological properties of emulsions may be discussed with respect to the disperse phase and the dispersion medium and the emulsifying agent.

The factors related to the disperse phase are the particle size distribution, phase-volume ratio and its viscosity. As the particle size of the disperse phase decreases, the viscosity increases. Wider particle size distribution may lower the viscosity. However wider particle size distribution is not always achieved. The viscosity is mainly dependent on mean particle size and the narrower distribution. When the volume of the disperse phase is as low as 0.05, the emulsion behaves like a Newtonian fluid and hence shows good flow property. Increase in volume of the disperse phase to reasonably high value in the emulsion, may result in more resistance to flow and may exhibit pseudoplastic flow characteristics. At sufficiently high concentration of the disperse phase, the flow becomes plastic. When the volume of the disperse phase exceeds 74% of the total volume of the emulsion, inversion of the emulsion (o/w may change to w/o) can occur with a marked change in viscosity.

In the case of dispersion medium, the factor that affects the flow is its own viscosity. However, the viscosity increases as the thickness of the film of the dispersion medium surrounding the particles of the disperse phase in a concentrated emulsion decreases to or below the range of 200Å to 100Å.

Emulsifying agent will affect the particle flocculation and interparticle attraction and hence the viscosity of the emulsion. The higher the proportion or concentration, the higher will be the viscosity of the emulsion.

Overall, the flow property of the emulsion should be so that it ensures the performance of the emulsion under the conditions of use or preparation. For example, spreadability of cosmetic products on application to skin, flowability through hypodermic needle during administration, and smooth pourability from a bottle or extrusion from a tube must be assured. Flow characteristics during milling, manufacturing, and bottling processes must also be satisfactory.

4. MICROMERITICS

Introduction

Whatever we consume be it drug or food, we take ultimately in small particulate sizes. All the materials in the universe, whether living or non-living, are made exclusively from small particles, scientifically expressing electrically neutral particles called atoms. Small and bigger molecules are formed from same or different atoms. When it comes to consumption, we use anything in reasonably small sized particles. When the size of the bigger particles are reduced to smaller particles, the properties especially (or sometimes astonishingly) the physical properties change. Nano-science assumes importance because of its size. There is, thus, a need to understand the science and technology of small particles and the study about this is called as micromeritics. It not always possible to get uniformly sized or shaped particles, when we reduce the size of bigger particles by some mechanical means. Hence, the distribution of particles about the mean is an important factor to be considered. This chapter deals with the size and size distribution and the scientific way of expressing them. It also deals with the methods to determine the size of particles and the properties derived because of size reduction and surface area increase.

Micromeritics

Mircromeritics is defined as the science and technology of small particles. This field has wider applications in pharmacy. They are:

1. The differentiation of solutions, colloids and suspensions depends upon the particle size of the dispersed phase only. In colloids, the particle size ranges from 1 nm to 0.5 μm and in suspensions, the particle size exceeds 0.5 μm.
2. The particle size in colloids and in suspensions decides their stability. The stability of the preparations decreases as the particle size increases and this leads to faster sedimentation.
3. The particle size of powder preparations is indirectly proportional to their surface area. The surface area of the given amount of powder gets increased as its particle size is decreased by size reduction. The relation between surface area and particle size is given by the expression.

$$S = \frac{6m}{d\rho} \qquad \text{... (1)}$$

where S = surface area

m = mass of the powder

d = diameter of the particles

ρ = density of the particles.

For a mass of 1 gram, assume that the diameter and the density have unit values, then the surface area is

$$S = \frac{6 \times 1}{1 \times 1} = 6$$

If the diameter is reduced 10 times the original value, the surface area is

$$S = \frac{6 \times 1}{0.1 \times 1} = 60$$

That is, the surface area is increased ten times the original surface area. The increased surface area enhances the contact surface with the solvent. This leads to increased rate of dissolution of drug powder. This, in turn, increases the absorption of the drug from the gastrointestinal tract and hence the bioavailability of the drug. The increased rate of bioavailability of drugs from gastrointestinal tract is as follows.

Tablets and capsules < big particles < micronized powder < suspensions < colloids < true solution

4. The particle size of the dispersed drug in ointment or suppositories affects its release characteristics from the dosage form to the skin or the mucous membrane.
5. The particle size decides the spreading ability and performance of some cosmetic preparations like dusting powder, face power, etc.
6. The size and shape of the particles in a powder decide its flow properties. The asymmetric particles have very poor flow properties. Hence granulation techniques are used to convert drug and the additive powders into symmetric spherical granules with good flow properties. This permits uniform supply of the drug powder from the hopper to the dies of the tablet machine. The tablets so produced will show uniform weights.

7. Particle size has a great effect on mixing of solids.
8. Process of separation of solids from fluids involves filtration and it is influenced by the particle size. Sedimentation also is influenced by particle size of powders.
9. Process factors such as loss as dust and explosion risk depend upon particle size of powders.
10. Extraction and drying are enhanced with smaller particle size of the material.
11. Adsorption capacity of a material will increase as the particle size decreases.

Particle size

For a symmetric particle like sphere, it is easy to describe the size by its diameter. i.e. size of a sphere can be described by its diameter. But most of the drug powders do not show symmetry in their shapes. Hence, the particle sizes of asymmetric particles are expressed in terms of *`equivalent spherical diameters'*. Equivalent spherical diameter is a method by which any parameter such as volume, surface area, projected diameter, or sedimentation rate of an asymmetric particle is equated to the volume, surface area, or sedimentation rate of a sphere and the diameter of the sphere is taken as the size of the asymmetric particle. Suppose the volume of an asymmetric particle is same as that of a spherical particle, then the size of the asymmetrical particle is taken as the size of the sphere and then the size of the asymmetric particle is given as the volume diameter. Similarly, the other diameters are given. This will be clear from the definitions given below. The various ways of expressing equivalent diameters are,

(i) Surface diameter (d_s): It is the diameter of a sphere having same surface area as that of the asymmetric particle in question.

(ii) Volume diameter (d_v): It is the diameter of a sphere having same volume as that of the asymmetric particle in question.

(iii) Projected diameter (d_p): It is the diameter of a sphere having same observed area as that of the asymmetric particle when viewed normal to its most stable plane by using a microscope.

(iv) Stoke's diameter or sedimentation diameter (d_{st}): It is the diameter of a sphere which undergoes sedimentation at the same rate as that of the asymmetric particle.

Particle size distribution

No powder (collection of particles) is monodisperse. That is, all the particles in a powder are not of the same size. It is only a polydisperse i.e. a mixture of different sized particles. Hence, it is necessary to know the size of particles and how many particles are present in each size range. Simply, distribution of different sized particles in a powder is called *particle size distribution*. From the data of particle size distribution, average particle size of the powder can be calculated.

Average particle size

The average particle size is given by the formula

$$\frac{\Sigma nd}{\Sigma n}$$

In the above method, only the total number and mean size of the particle have been considered to express the average particle size. The expression of average particle size can further be extended to take into account the surface and the volume of the particles. Edmundson has derived a general equation to express the average particle size. It is given as

$$d_{mean} = \left(\frac{\Sigma nd^{p+f}}{\Sigma nd^{f}}\right)^{1/p}$$

where $n =$ number of particles in each size range whose mid point is d which is one of the equivalent diameters.

$p =$ an index related to size of an individual particle $p = 1, p = 2, or\ p = 3$ which expresses particle length, surface or volume respectively. The value of the index p also decides whether the mean is arithmetic, geometric or harmonic. If the value of p is positive, the mean is *arithmetic*, if p is zero, the mean is *geometric,* and if p is negative, the mean is *harmonic.*

For a collection of particles, the frequency with which a particle in certain size range occurs is expressed by nd^f in which f is called frequency index which has values 0,1,2 or 3. Thus the size frequency distribution is expressed in terms of total number or length or surface or volume of the particles respectively.

Statistical diameters

Size index (p)	Frequency index (f)	Edumundson equation $d_{mean} = \left(\frac{\Sigma\, nd^{p+f}}{\Sigma\, nd^{f}}\right)^{1/p}$	Type of mean	Mean diameter is based on
1	0	$\Sigma nd/\Sigma n$	Arithmetic	Length number mean (d_{ln})
2	0	$\sqrt{\frac{\Sigma\, nd^2}{\Sigma\, n}}$	Arithmetic	Surface number mean (d_{sn})
3	0	$\sqrt{\frac{\Sigma\, nd^3}{\Sigma\, n}}$	Arithmetic	Volume number mean (d_{vn})
1	1	$\frac{\Sigma\, nd^2}{\Sigma\, nd}$	Arithmetic	Length weighted mean
1	2	$\frac{\Sigma\, nd^3}{\Sigma\, nd^2}$	Arithmetic	Surface weighted mean
1	3	$\frac{\Sigma\, nd^4}{\Sigma\, nd^3}$	Arithmetic	Volume weight mean

Size index $p = 1$ means length is considered as a size parameter

Size index $p = 2$ means surface is considered as a size parameter

Size index $p = 3$ means volume is considered as a size parameter

Frequency index $f = 0$ means number is considered as a frequency parameter

Frequency index $f = 1$ means length is considered as a frequency parameter

Frequency index $f = 2$ means surface is considered as a frequency parameter

Size distribution is often complex. In a sample of powder, different sized particles (i.e. polydisperse) can be found. Hence, it may be necessary to classify the successive size ranges. The distribution can be represented by a bar graph or histogram in which the bars represent the size range and the heights of the bars represent the frequency of occurrence of particular size range. Any given powder is polydisperse and it may be quantified by two ways.

1. Number of particles present in each size range (found out by microscopy)
2. Weight of particles present in each size range (found out by sedimentation or sieving techniques)

Suppose we find the number of particles in each size range using a microscope and the data obtained from such a determination is presented in table, 1.

Table 1. Particle Size Distribution Data

Size range in μm	Mean size d in μm	Number of particles in each size range (n) obtained by microscopy (frequency)
2 – 4	3	10
4 – 6	5	26
6 – 8	7	58
8 – 10	9	110
10 – 12	11	56
12 – 14	13	24
14 – 16	15	9
		293

If we want to compare these values with those of a successive batch or a second batch of the same material, the average or mean diameter obtained by calculation may not serve as a better basis for comparison of the two batches. Hence, with these values, a histogram may be obtained by plotting each size range against the frequency of occurrence of particles (Fig. 1). A smooth curve drawn through the midpoints of the top of the bars (midpoints represent the average size or the middle value of the respective size range) yields a normal distribution curve (as shown in Fig.1). The curve obtained is often termed as *frequency distribution curve.*

Every time, we need not go for histogram (unless otherwise needed). A frequency distribution curve will serve the purpose for the number or weight distribution.

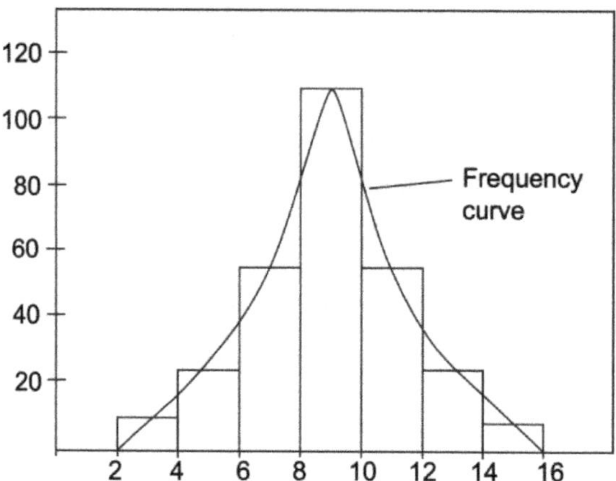

Fig. 4.1 Histogram with frequency curve

A size frequency curve provides a clear visible representation of the distribution of particles in a powder whereas the expression of size in terms of average diameter cannot give such a clear expression. Two powders having the same average diameter may not have the same frequency distribution. From such plots, we can make out the particle size which occurs more frequently and that size is called the *mode* of the sample. If the number of particles counted is considerably more, mean size can be plotted against **% frequency instead of frequency**. Usually the mean size (of each size range) is plotted against % frequency.

A polydisperse powder is said to have normal distribution if the data plotted show a typical bell shaped curve (frequency curve shown in Fig. 4.1). In this one half of the curve is super-imposable with another half, that is, the distribution of particles is symmetric around the mean and hence, it is termed as *normal distribution curve*. In this case *mode* and mean (*average size)* are same. The standard deviation (σ) is the indication of the distribution about the mean. The *standard deviation* is defined as the root-mean square deviation about the mean. In a normal distribution, 68% of the particles lie within $\pm 1\sigma$ from the mean, 95% of the particles lie within $\pm 2\sigma$ from the mean and 99.7% lie within $\pm 3\sigma$ from the mean. Most of the powders (i.e after size reduction) do not show this distribution.

Most particulate material cannot be described by a normal distribution curve since the particle size distribution of most of the pharmaceutical powders tends to be asymmetric or skewed. Such skewed distribution may be obtained from number distribution data or weight distribution data given in Table.2 (refer Fig. 4.2 and 4.4).

The particle size data distribution of a given powder can be scientifically represented as follows in Table 2.

1	2	3	4	5	6	7	8
Size range μm	Mean size (d)	No. of particles in each size range (n)	% Frequency (number)	Cumalitive % frequency under size (number)	$n \times d^3$ (Weight)	Percent frequency (weight)	Cumalitive % frequency under size (weight)
1 – 3	2.0	4	1	1	32	0.01	0.01
3– 5	4.0	62	15.5	16.5	3968	1.53	1.54
5 - 7	6.0	132	33	48.5	28512	10.98	12.52
7 – 9	8.0	94	23.5	73	48128	18.53	31.05
9 – 11	10.0	58	14.5	87.5	58000	22.34	53.39
11 – 13	12.0	30	7.5	95	51840	19.97	73.36
13 – 15	14.0	12	3	98	32928	12.68	86.04
15 – 17	16.0	6	1.5	99.5	24576	9.46	95.5
17 - 19	18.0	2	0.5	100	11664	4.49	99.99
Total		400	100		259648	99.99	

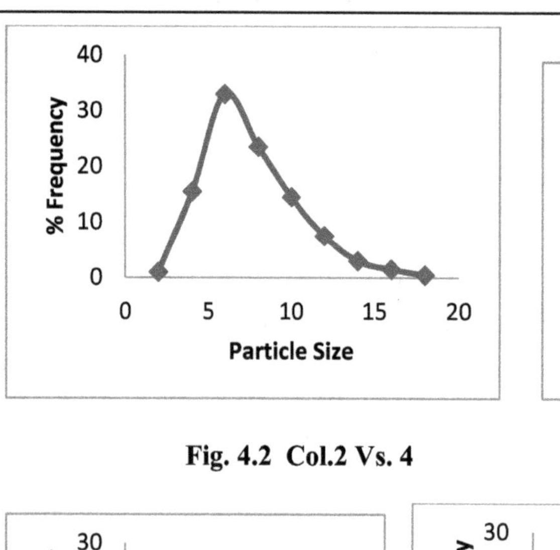

Fig. 4.2 Col.2 Vs. 4

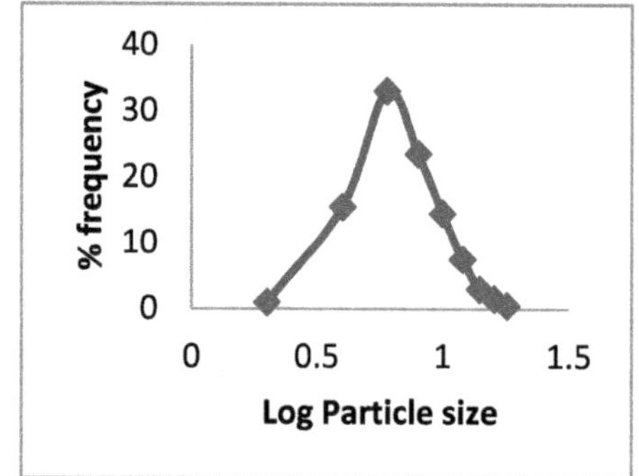

Fig. 4.3

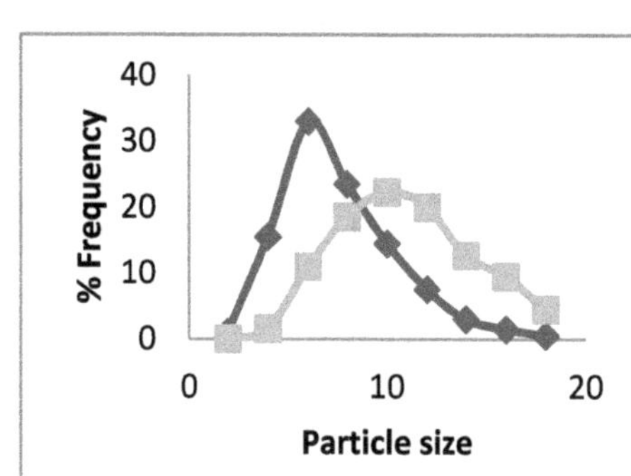

Fig. 4.4 Col 2 Vs 7

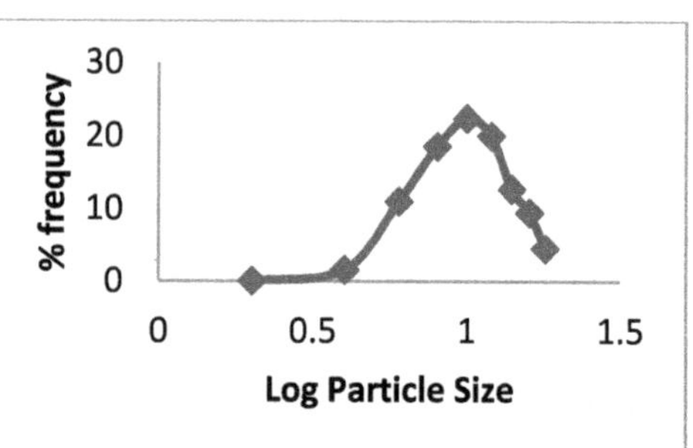

Fig. 4.5

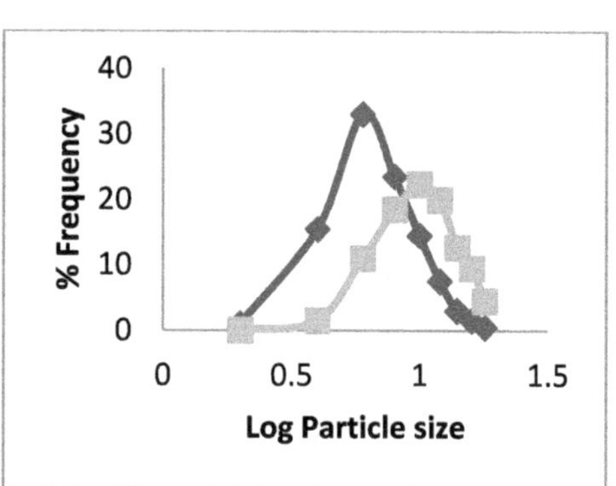

Fig. 4.6 % frequency in number

Fig. 4.7 % frequency in weight

In skewed or asymmetric distribution, the mode and mean are different. Most asymmetric size distribution curves relating to powders can be converted into symmetrical curves by plotting logarithm of the size against percent (%) frequency (either number or weight) i.e. a nearly bell shaped curve can be obtained. Frequently such a curve is called *log normal distribution curve*

(Fig: 4.3 and 4.5.) For plotting, a semi-log paper can be used if arithmetic values are used instead of logarithmic values. The symmetrical shape of the curve thus obtained by plotting the logarithm of size versus the frequency allows for simplified mathematical analysis. Skewed and log-normal distribution curves can be shown together for comparison's sake as sown in figures 4.6 and 4.7. one can observe that all the figures provide a clear representation of the distribution of particles in a powder. It may be noted that there is significant differences in the two distributions i.e. the number and weight distribution, though they relate to the same sample. For example, only 12.5 % of the sample by number is greater than 10 µm whereas the weight for the same sample accounts for about 46.6 % of the total weight of the particles. This is evident from the Fig. 4.8. It can also be clearly noted from the Table 2 by looking at the column 4 and 7.

Plotting either the cumulative percent oversize or undersize against the particle size gives a sigmoidal curve with the mode being at the greatest slope as shown in Fig. 4.8

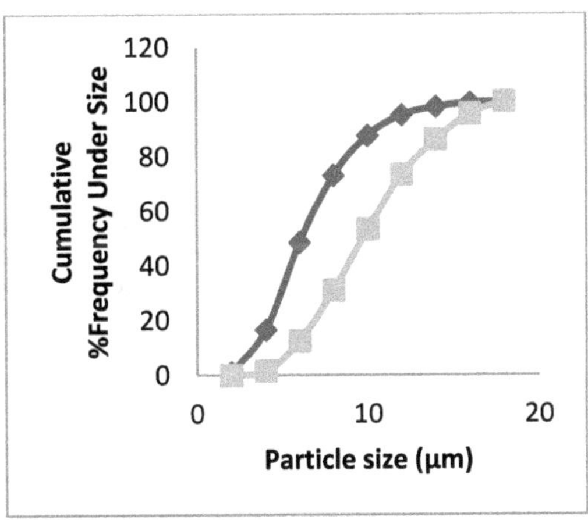

Fig. 4.8 Col 2 Vs 5 and 8

A log normal distribution has several properties of interest. When the logarithm of the particle size is plotted against the cumulative percent frequency on a probability scale or on probit values, a linear relationship can be obtained (Fig. 4.9). Such a linear plot can be used to characterize a log-normal distribution curve by means of two parameters – the slope of the line and the reference point. Using these two parameters, one can reproduce Fig. 4.9 and by working back, can come up with a good approximation of Fig 4.6, 4.7 and 4.8. The reference point is the logarithm of particle size equivalent to 50% on probability scale or probit scale of 50% size. This 50% size is known as geometric mean diameter. The geometric mean distribution is represented as d_g for number distribution data and for weight distribution, it is represented as d′g). The slope gives the geometric standard deviation (σ_g) and it is invariably same for number and weight distribution.

Number and weight distribution

Number distribution can be obtained by counting the particles in a sample of powder using a microscope. For weight distribution, sieving or sedimentation technique can be used. However, it it will be more convenient for our consideration if the number distribution data obtained by microscope is used for weight distribution by converting the number distribution into weight distribution.

Two approaches are available for the conversion of number distribution into weight distribution.

First approach is by using the formula nd^3 provided the general shape and density of the particles are independent of the size range of the particles in the powder.

The second approach is by using one of the Hatch-Choate equations provided the distribution is log-normal. With the use of Hatch-Choate equations, it is possible to convert number distribution into weight distribution and *vice versa*. With the use of Hatch-Choate equations, other statistical parameters can be calculated such as length-number mean, surface-number mean, volume-number mean, volume-surface mean, and weight –moment mean using geometric mean diameter and geometric standard deviation (either of number distribution or of weight distribution). In order to get the geometric mean diameter and geometric standard deviation, the log of mean size is plotted against the *probit values* (see Addendum – page 234) of cumulative percent frequency undersize (number and weight) are obtained using the data given in table 2, and for convenience sake, the data may be presented separately in the following table 3.

Table. 3

Mean size	Log of mean size	Cumulative % frequency under size (number)	Probit values for cumulative % frequency undersize (number)	Cumulative % frequency under size (weight)	Probit values for cumulative % frequency undersize (weight)
2	0.3010	1	2.67	0.01	-
4	0.6020	16.5	4.01	1.54	2.9
6	0.7781	49.5	4.97	12.52	3.82
8	0.9031	73.0	5.61	31.05	4.50
10	1.0000	87.5	6.13	53.39	5.08
12	1.0791	95.0	6.64	73.36	5.61
14	1.1461	98.0	7.05	86.04	6.08
16	1.2041	99.5	7.58	95.5	6.64
18	1.2552	100	8.09	99.99	8.09

By plotting the log mean size on x axis against empirical probit values for cumulative percentage frequency undersize (number) on y axis using an ordinary arithemtic graph paper as shown in Fig. 4.9, one obtains a straight line. The line so obtained may be characterized by two parameters that are the slope of the line and the reference point. The reference point is the logarithm of the particle size equivalent to 50% on the probit scale which is called *geometric mean diameter*. In this case, value of log particle size corresponding to 50% probit value (5.0) for number distribution is 0.79. The antilog of 0.79 is 6.16 μm which is the *geometric mean diameter* (d_g) of the powder. If the geometric mean diameter is derived from the similar type of graph using weight distribution, the geometric mean diameter of the powder is designated as d'_g and the value comes out to be 9.77 μm (antilog of 0.99) because on 50% probit value, the log particle size is 0.99 in the present example. Both the number and weight distribution are shown in Fig. 4.9

using same graph paper. In the present example, the 16% under size (equal to 4.0 on probit value) for number distribution is 0.61 in log value and the antilog for this value is 4.07 μm. For weight distribution, the 16% under size is 6.45 μm (the antilog of 0.81)

For number distribution 50% size

For 50% size dg = 6.16 μm (antilog of 0.79)

For weight distribution 50% size

For 50% weight d'g = 9.77 μm (antilog of 0.99)

$$\sigma_g = \frac{50\%\ size}{16\%\ undersize} = \frac{6.16}{4.07}\ (\text{or})\ \frac{9.77}{6.45} = 1.51\ \mu m$$

4.07 is the antilog of 0.61 and 6.45 is the antilog of 0.81 for 16% undersize of number and weight distribution respectively).

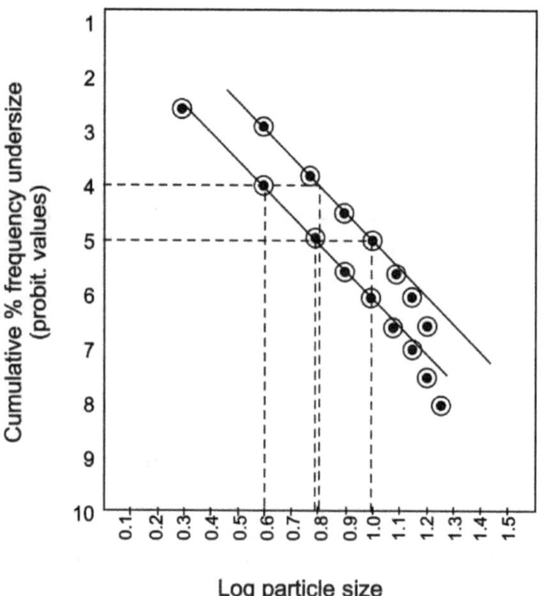

Fig. 4.9

The geometric standard deviation $\sigma_g = \frac{84\%\ \text{undersize or}\ 16\%\ \text{oversize}}{50\%\ \text{size}}$

$$\text{or, } \frac{50\%\ \text{size}}{16\%\ \text{undersize or}\ 84\%\ \text{oversize}}$$

From the data obtained,

$$\sigma_g = \frac{\text{50\% size}}{\text{16\% undersize}} = \frac{6.16}{4.07} = 1.51\ \mu\text{m}$$

Using the weight distribution data, the geometric standard deviation (σ_g) also comes out to be $1.51\,\mu\text{m}$ (as for number distribution) in the present example.

Particle Number (N)

It is defined as the number of particles per unit weight.

Assume the particles of a powder are spherical. Then, the volume of a single particle is $\pi d_{vn}^3/6$ where d_{vn} is the mean diameter based on volume and number. The mass of the particle is $\pi d_{vn}^3 \rho/6$ (i.e. mass = volume × density) where ρ is density of the particle.

Number of particles per gram (N)

$$= \frac{\text{1 gm of the powder}}{\text{Mass of one particle}} = 6/\pi d_{vn}^3 \rho \qquad \ldots(6)$$

Thus if mean volume number of a powder and density are known, the number of particles per gram can be calculated.

Determination of particle size

Frequently, particle size measurements are made along with separation of the powder into fractions based on size. The various methods employed for measurement, classification, or the fractionation of powder particles involve direct and indirect techniques. In direct methods, the actual dimensions of the particles are made. Microscopy and sieving methods are the direct methods which use calibration scale. Indirect methods make use of some characteristic of the particle that can be related to particle size, such as sedimentation rates, particle volume, etc.

1. Microscopic technique
2. Sieving technique
3. Sedimentation technique
4. Coulter counter (electrical method) technique
5. Low angle light scattering technique

1. Microscopic Technique

An ordinary compound microscope is used for determination. First of all, an eye piece micrometer which may be square or linear type should be calibrated. For calibration a standard stage micrometer is used. In this `one millimeter is divided into 100 equal divisions and hence each division is equal to 10 μ. The eye piece micrometer which is linear consists of 100 divisions. Calibration is undertaken to find out the measure of each division using the standard micrometer. After calibration, the eye piece micrometer is used for particle size determination.

A suspension (diluted) of the powder particles whose sizes are to be determined is prepared in a liquid vehicle in which it is insoluble. If it is slightly soluble, a saturated solution of the powder can be used for the preparation of the suspension. A drop of the suspension is mounted on a slide and observed under the microscope. About 300 particles are measured with the help of the eye piece micrometer. All the particles in a field should be counted. The data may be presented as follows.

S.No.	Diameter of the particles
1	X_1
2	X_2
.	
.	
n	X_n

The above data may be rearranged as follows:

Size range	mid point	No. of particles in each size range
...	...	...
...	...	...
...	...	...

The data can be scientifically represented as size-frequency distribution curve as described earlier. From the data, the average particle size can be found out. Particles in the size range of 0.2 μm to about 100 μm can be measured by this technique.

Disadvantages

1. The diameter of the particles represents two dimensions only i.e. length and breadth and not the depth.
2. At least 300 to 500 particles should be counted to get a reliable data and hence the method is tedious.

Advantages

The presence of agglomerates can easily be detected and avoided.

Improvements

1. The field viewed through the microscope can be projected for easy counting and measurement of the particles.
2. The field of the microscope can be photographed for measurement of the particles.
3. Particles may be counted with electronic scanners to avoid the strain of visual observation.
4. A double image microscope may be used. In this, the image of the particle is split until the two images are just separated using a calibrated image splitting device. The adjustment needed for this gives the particle diameter.
5. By using an electron microscope, particles from 1 Å to 1μm can also be measured.

2. Sieving Technique

A series of standard sieves are stacked one above the other so that sieves with larger pore size (less sieve numbers) occupy top portion followed by sieves of decreasing pore sizes (larger sieve numbers) towards the bottom. (The sieve number indicates the number of pores per linear inch, Suppose, the sieve number is 10, it indicates that it contains 10 pores (meshes) per linear inch or 100 pores per square inch)

Sieve apertures (which represent the actual or effective pore sizes) ranging from 90μm down to as low as 5μm are available. A definite mass of the sample is placed on the top sieve and the whole set-up is shaken mechanically for a definite period of time. The powder remaining on each sieve after the agitation is over, is collected separately and weighted. The data are summarized as follows.

S. No.	Sieve No.	Sieve aperture size μm	Weight of powder detained in each sieve
...	...	...	...
...	...	...	...

The geometric mean diameter (d'_g and standard deviation (σ'_g can be obtained by the method described earlier.

Disadvantages

Sieving errors may occur due to sieve loading and duration and intensity of agitation. Sieving may also cause attrition of granular pharmaceutical material (this produces size reduction). Hence enough care should be exercised to avoid errors introduced due to sieving conditions.

Depending upon the sieve number, powder particles may be classified as follows:

Sieve number (All the particles passes through)	Sieve Number Not more than 40% of powder pass through	Grade of the powder
10	44	Coarse powder
22	60	Moderately coarse powder
44	85	Moderately fine powder
85	-	Fine powder
120	-	Very fine powder

3. Sedimentation technique

This may be carried out by using an ***Andreasen pipette*** (Fig. 4.9). It consists of a 550 ml vessel containing a 10 ml pipette sealed into a ground glass stopper. When the pipette is in its place in the cylinder, the lower tip is 20 cm below the surface of the suspension.

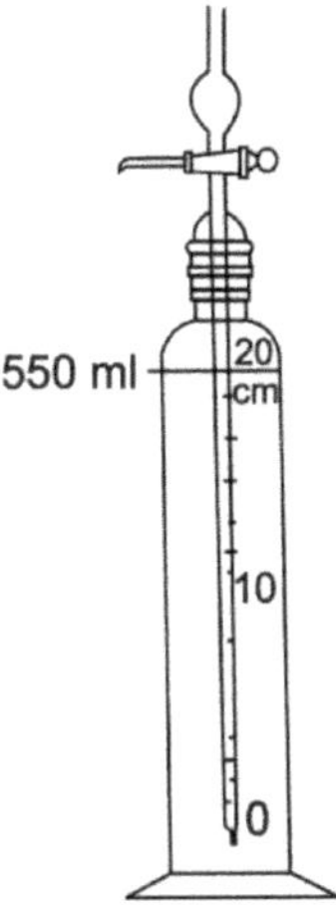

Fig. 4.9 Andreasen apparatus

For analysis, 1 to 2% suspension of powder particles in a medium containing a suitable deflocculating agent (to separate any aggregate) is introduced into the vessel upto the mark 20 cm and that represents a total volume of 550 ml. The vessel is stoppered and shaken to distribute the particles uniformly within the medium. Having placed the pipette securely in its place, the vessel is clamped in a constant temperature bath. At various time intervals 10 ml samples are withdrawn into a previously weighed china dish every time. Each sample is evaporated and weighed separately and necessary correction is made for the deflocculating agent.

The particle diameter corresponding to the various time period is calculated as follows by using Stoke's equation:

$$v = \frac{d_{st}^2(\rho - \rho_1)g}{18\eta_l} \qquad \text{... (7)}$$

where v = rate of sedimentation

d_{st} = sedimentation diameter of the particle i.e. Stoke's diameter

ρ_s = density of the powder

ρ_l = density of the medium

g = acceleration due to gravity

η_l = viscosity of the medium

The rate of sedimentation is

$$v = \frac{h}{t} \qquad \text{... (8)}$$

Where, h is the distance of the fall of particles in time t

On substitution for v and rearrangement for d_{st}, the equation becomes:

$$d_{st} = \sqrt{\frac{18\eta_l h}{(\rho_s - \rho_l)gt}} \qquad \text{...(9)}$$

Substituting appropriate values in the equation (9), d_{st} of particles at different time intervals can be calculated.

To apply Stoke's law, flow of dispersion medium around the particle as it sediments should be laminar or streamline. Whether the flow is laminar or turbulent is indicated by Reynold's number (R_e)

$$R_e = \frac{vd\rho_l}{\eta_l} \qquad \text{... (10)}$$

Now $v = \frac{R_e}{d}\frac{\eta_l}{\rho_l}$

Thus $\frac{R_e}{d}\frac{\eta_l}{\rho_l} = \frac{d^2(\rho_s - \rho_l)g}{18\,\eta_l}$

$$d^3 = \frac{18R_e\eta_l^2}{(\rho_s - \rho_l)\rho_l g} \qquad \text{... (18)}$$

This expression gives maximum diameter where sedimentation rate is governed by Stoke's law and the Reynold's number does not exceed 0.2.

The results are tabulated as follows

S. No.	Time period in minutes (t)	d_{st} at t	Weight of powder collected at different time intervals
...	...	...	...
...	...	...	...
...	...	...	...

From the data, various graphs needed may be obtained. Then the geometric mean diameter (d'_g) and standard deviation (σ'_g) for this weight distribution can also be calculated.

The improved technique of sedmimentation method is the centrifugal method. When the particles are very small, normal sedimentation is very slow. Hence centrifugal force is used to accelerate sedimentation instead of gravitational sedimentation. The particle size of the sediment at different time intervals is monitored by turbidometric method. In this, a beam of light is passed through the suspension. Some of the light is scattered and can be measured and from this the surface area of the particles can be calculated. Using appropriate equations, the particle size can be found. This method has a special advantage because the suspension is not disturbed as in pipette sampling.

4. Coulter counter method (Electrical method to measure particle volume)

A Coulter consists of the following parts as shown in Fig. 4.10.

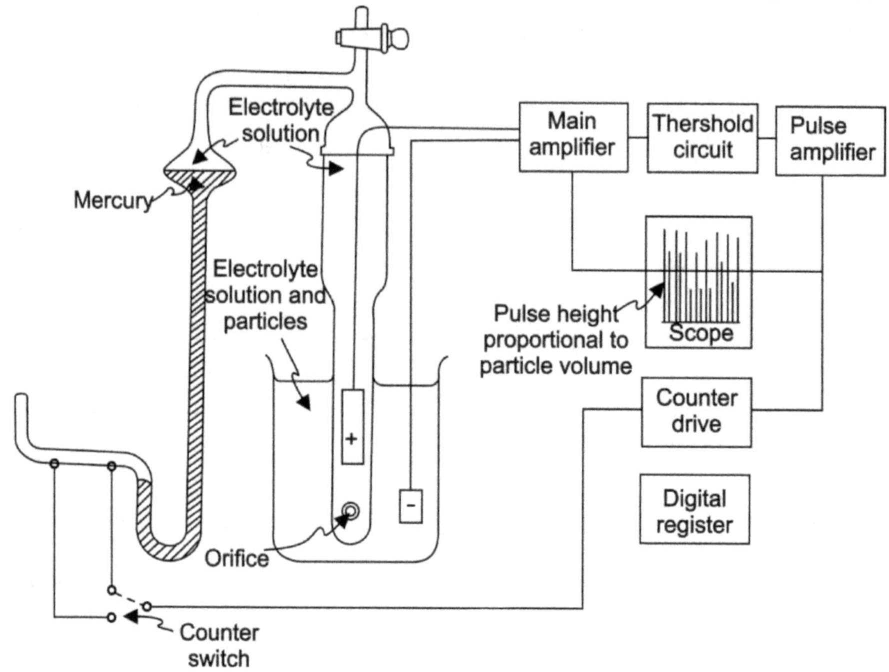

Fig. 4.10 Coulter current method

It consists of two electrodes of which one is dipped into a vessel containing the electrolyte and the particles and the other is dipped in the electrolyte solution in a tube which in turn is dipped into the vessel. The tube and the vessel are connected through an orifice. The terminals are connected to an amplifier. The tube is connected to the counter device via mercury in a tube.

A known volume of dilute suspension in an electrolyte solution is kept in the vessel. The dispersion is pumped through the orifice into the tube. The suspension should be so dilute that at a time only one particle passes through the orifice. A constant voltage is applied across the electrodes. As the particle travels through the orifice, it displaces its own volume of the electrolyte and this results in an increased resistance between the two electrodes. The change in resistance which is related to particle volume causes a voltage pulse. The pulse is amplified and fed to an oscilloscope (pulse height analyzer) calibrated in terms of particle size.

To avoid overcrowding, the electronic circuit is provided with a threshold selector which can be set for any particle size range. Suppose we set the instrument for the particle size range from 10 μm to 100 μm the instrument will detect only those particles in that range. A typical print out will have the following data.

Number of particles counted	Pulse height	Particle size
...	...	...
...	...	...
...	...	...

Using this instrument, all the particles can be counted. The instrument is capable of counting at the rate of 4000 particles per second approximately. The instrument is also used to find out particulate contamination in parenteral solution as per USP specifications.

From the pulse height, volume distribution can be obtained and this can be converted to weight distribution.

The choice of the method for particle size analysis is summarised as follows:

Method	Size range
Sieving	10 μm to 10,000 μm
Optical microscope	1 μm to 100 μm
Electron microscope	1Å to 1 μm
Sedimentation	1 μm to 660 μm
Ultracentrifuge	10 Å to 1 μm
Coulter counter	0.5 μm to 1000 μm

5. Low angle Laser Light Scattering Technique

In this Laser diffraction principle (more correctly - low angle laser light scattering - LALLS) particle size is measured accurately and precisely. Particles are irregular in shape and hence their size can vary greatly depending upon chosen dimension for measurement and the results vary depending upon different techniques of measurement. LALLS technique is speedy, easy and reproducible for particle size determination. Particles ranging from 0.5 μm to 3500 μm can be measured. A wide range of samples including dry powders, liquid suspension, aerosols, emulsions, particulate contaminant in injections can be anaylsed. Small amount of samples (10 mg) is enough. The technique is non - destructive.

No calibration against a standard is necessary. The instrument used for this purpose is called Malveran Master sizer.

Particle shape

Particle shape affects the flow characteristics and packing properties of a powder.

A sphere has minimum surface area per unit volume. The more asymmetric the particle becomes, the greater is the surface area per unit volume. Hence it may be necessary to know the extent of asymmetry in a particle.

The surface area or volume of a sphere is given by

$$\text{Surface area} = \pi d^2 \qquad \text{... (12)}$$

$$\text{Volume} = \frac{\pi d^3}{6} \qquad \text{... (13)}$$

To estimate the surface area or volume of an asymmetric particle, we must choose a diameter that relates this to the surface area or the volume of a sphere through a correction factor.

Suppose we obtain the size of a particle microscopically, then the size is given in terms of diameter as projected diameter d_p for the particle. Now the square and cube of this chosen diameter (i.e d_p) are proportional to the surface area and volume respectively. Making use of proportionality constant, we can write.

$$\text{Surface area} = \alpha_s\, d_p^2 = \pi\, d_s^2$$

where α_s is the surface area factor and d_s is the equivalent surface diameter (i.e spherical particle)

Then, $\alpha_s = \frac{\pi d_s^2}{d_p^2} = 3.142$

Thus, the shape factor α_s is the ratio of one diameter to another.

For volume, we can write

Volume = $\alpha_v \, d_p^3 = \frac{\pi d_v^3}{6}$

Where α_v is the volume factor and d_v is the equivalent volume diameter

$$\text{Then, } \alpha_v = \frac{\pi d_v^2}{d_p^3 .6} = 0.524 \qquad \text{... (14)}$$

Each and every particle has its own volume and shape factors.

Taking the ratio of surface area factor and volume factor, we get

$$\frac{\alpha_s}{\alpha_v} = \frac{\pi d_s^2 \, d_p^3 \, 6}{d_p^2 \, \pi d_v^3}$$

If the particle is spherical

$$\frac{\alpha_s}{\alpha_v} = 6$$

(since all the other terms get cancelled for a spherical particle)

If this ratio (α_s / α_v) exceeds 6, then the particle deviates from being a sphere and it can be said, the more this ratio exceeds this minimum value of 6, the more asymmetric the particle becomes.

Specific surface

Specific surface is defined as the surface area per unit volume (S_v) or per unit weight (S_w)

Taking into account, the surface area factor and volume factor for n number of asymmetric particles, specific surface per unit volume is

$$S_V = \frac{\text{Surface area of } n \text{ particles}}{\text{volume of } n \text{ particles}}$$

$$= \frac{n \, \alpha_s d^2}{n \, \alpha_v d^3} = \frac{\alpha_s}{\alpha_v d}$$

Specific surface area per unit weight is

$$S_W = \frac{\text{Surface area of } n \text{ particles}}{\text{Volume of } n \text{ particles } \times \text{density}}$$

$$S_w = \frac{n\,\alpha_s d^2}{n\,\alpha_v d^3\,\rho}$$

where $\rho =$ true density of the particle

$$= \frac{\alpha_s}{\alpha_v\, d\rho}$$

or $$S_w = \frac{S_v}{\rho} \quad \text{(where } S_v = (\frac{\alpha_s}{\alpha_v d})\text{)} \qquad \text{... (15)}$$

Defining the dimension as d_{vs} which is volume surface diameter characteristics of specific surface, the above equation is written as

$$S_w = \frac{\alpha_s}{\alpha_v d_{vs}\,\rho} \qquad \text{... (16)}$$

For spherical particles

$$S_w = \frac{6}{d_{vs}\,\rho} \text{ (since } \frac{\alpha_s}{\alpha_v} = 6 \text{ for spherical particles)}$$

8.1. Determination of surface area of powders

The surface area of a powder can be derived indirectly from the size and size distribution obtained by the methods (such as microscopy, sieving, sedimentation and volume determined by Coulter counter) already described. Direct calculation of surface area may be done using two methods. They are the adsorption and air permeability methods.

1. Adsorption method

In this method, the amount of solute in solution or a gas that is adsorbed onto a sample of powder to form a monolayer is found out and from this data, surface area of the powder may be determined.

(a) By using a solute which forms a monolayer: This involves the adsorption of a solute from solution onto the surface of a powder (i.e. adsorbent)

Methanolic solution of stearic acid is first prepared. Stearic acid being a linear molecule, the molecules get adsorbed on solid surface (i.e. on powder surface) as a monolayer. The method is applicable to adsorbent powders insoluble in methanol.

A known amount of adsorbent powder is treated with excess amount of methanolic solution of stearic acid. The contents are stirred. After one hour or after ensuring that adsorption has attained equilibrium, it is filtered. The filtrate contains unadsorbed stearic acid. It is estimated by titrating with a standard solution of sodium hydroxide. A blank tritration is performed to find out the amount of stearic acid originally present in the solution. The difference between these values gives the amount of stearic acid adsorbed by the quantity of the powder added. From this value, the amount of stearic acid adsorbed per gram of the material can be calculated. Assume this to be `x' grams. The number of molecules present in 1 gram mole of stearic acid (i.e. 284 gm) is given by Avogadro's number, 6.0223×10^{23}. From these data it is quite simple to find out what will be the number of molecules present in x grams of stearic acid. Let the number of molecules present in x grams be n and since one molecule of stearic acid occupies an area of 20.46×10^{-16} sq. cm., the total surface area of stearic acid molecules in x grams is $n \times 20.46 \times 10^{-16}$ sq. cm. This gives the specific surface. The specific surface may also be expressed in square meters per gram.

(b) By using adsorption of gas on powder: For this an instrument called *Quantasorb* may be used. The powder whose surface area is to be determined is introduced into a cell in the instrument and nitrogen which is the adsorbate gas and helium which is an inert gas and not adsorbed are passed through the powder in the cell. A thermal conductivity detector measures the amount of nitrogen adsorbed at every equilibrium pressure and a bell shaped curve is obtained on a strip-chart recorder. The signal height gives the rate of adsorption of nitrogen gas and the area under the curve provides the amount of gas adsorbed on the powder sample.

The volume of nitrogen gas V_m in cm^3 adsorbed by 1 gram of the powder when the monolayer is complete is given by BET equation as.

$$\frac{p}{V(p_o - p)} = \frac{1}{V_m b} + \frac{(b-1)p}{V_m b p_o} \quad \text{... (17)}$$

where v = volume of gas in cm^3 adsorbed per gram of powder at pressure p

p_o = saturated vapour pressure of liquified nitrogen at the temperature of the experiment.

b = a constant and it gives the difference between the heat of adsorption and the heat of liquefaction of the nitrogen gas.

A plot of $p/V(p_o - p)$ against p/p_o ordinarily yields a straight line. The slope and intercept yield the values b and v respectively (Fig. 4.11).

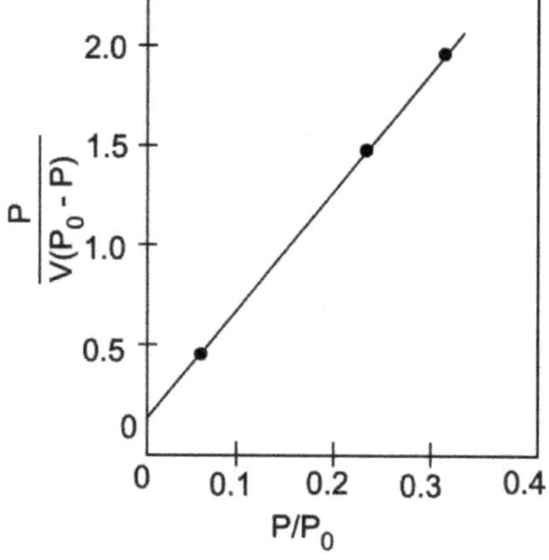

Fig. 4.11

The specific surface of the powder is obtained by applying the equation given below

$$S_w = \frac{A_m N}{M/\rho} \times V_m$$

where $\frac{M}{\rho}$ = molar volume of the gas at N.T.P.

N = Avogadro's number 6.02×10^{23}

A_m = area of a single close packed gas molecule adsorbed as a monolayer on the surface of the powder particles. For nitrogen the value is $16.2 \times 10^{-16} cm^2$.

Quantasorb may be used to determine the true density of powders and to obtain pore size and pore volume distributions for porous materials.

2.Air permeability method

Surface area determination by air permeability method can be carried out with an instrument called *Fisher subsieve sizer*. The instrument is shown in Fig. 4.12.

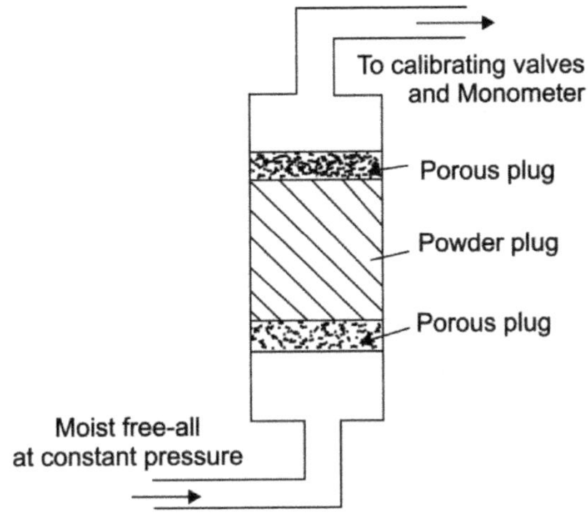

Fig. 4.12 Fisher Subsieve Sizer

A plug of powder is considered to have a series of capillaries whose diameter is related to average particle size. According to Poiseuille's equation.

$$v = \frac{\pi d^4 \Delta pt}{8l\eta}$$

where v is the volume of air flowing through a capillary of internal diameter d and length l in t seconds under a pressure difference of Δp The viscosity of the fluid (air) is η poise.

When the air is allowed to pass through the plug of a compacted powder, resistance to the flow of air occurs. This resistance is related to the surface area of the powder. As per Kozency-Carman equation derived from Poiseuille's equation.

$$v = \frac{A}{\eta S_w^2} \frac{\Delta pt}{kl} \frac{\varepsilon^3}{(1-\varepsilon)^2}$$

where A = cross sectional area of the plug.

k = a constant (usually 5.0 ± 0.5)

ε = porosity

From the values of A, k, ε (See under porosity of powders), ΔP (which is obtained from the manometer, η (the visocity of the fluid air), v (the volume of the air that flowed in time t), and the specific surface S_w can be calculated.

This method is widely used to control batch to batch variations in specific surface of powders. As the porosity of powder decreases, surface area of the powder is also decreased.

Derived properties of powders

The size *distribution* and the *surface area* are the two fundamental properties of the powders. Based upon these two properties, there are a number of derived properties. They are as follows.

Dissolution and dissolution rate

Dissolution and dissolution rate are a direct property of surface area increase due to size reduction.

Densities of powders

(a) Bulk density: It is the ratio between a given mass of a powder and its bulk volume.

$$\text{Bulk density} = \frac{\text{Mass of a powder}}{\text{Bulk volume of the powder}}$$

A given quantity of the powder is transferred to a measuring cylinder and is tapped mechanically either manually or using some tapping device till a constant volume is obtained. This volume is the bulk volume (v) and it includes the true volume of the powder and the void space among the powder particles. A true volume refers to the volume of solid particles (or a powder) excluding all spaces greater than molecular size.

A given pack of powder has air spaces between the particles. This air space is called void space or void volume (Fig. 4.13). Thus, the bulk volume is the true volume of the powder plus the void volume (void volume refers to the interparticulte void spaces which are filled by air)..

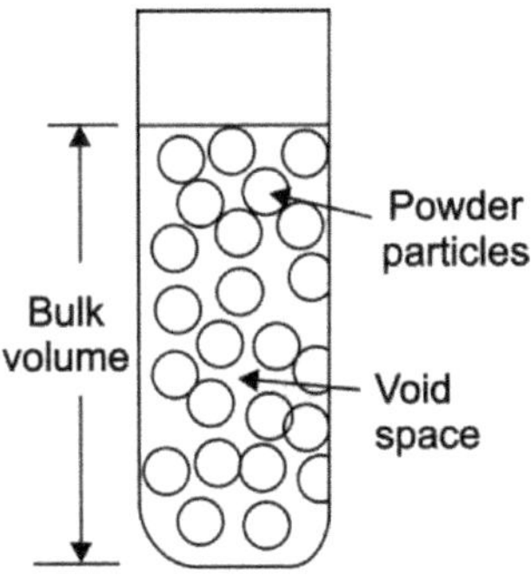

Fig. 4.13

(b) True density: The ratio between a given mass of a powder and its true volume (v) is called true density.

True volume = bulk volume – void volume

The true density of a powder can be determined as follows:

(i) Liquid displacement method: A 25cc standard flask may be used for the determination of true volume. Some amount of powder, whose true density is to be found out, is added into the flask and the weight is found out. Now a liquid in which the powder is insoluble is added to occupy the void spaces within the powder until the powder and liquid together occupy the volume i.e 25cc. Again it is weighed. Empty the contents of the flask and add only the liquid upto the 25cc mark and weigh it. The calculation may be carried out as given below.

Weight of the empty bottle = a grams

Weight of the bottle + liquid = b grams

Weight of the bottle + powder = c grams

Weight of the bottle + liquid + powder = d grams

The weight of the powder = $c - a$ grams

Density of the liquid $(\rho) = \frac{b-a}{25}$

True density $= \frac{\text{weight of the powder}}{\text{true volume}}$

$$= \frac{c-a}{25-\left(\frac{d-c}{\rho}\right)}$$

$$\text{Or } \frac{c-a}{\left(\frac{(b-a)}{\rho}\right)-\left(\frac{d-c}{\rho}\right)}$$

A pycnometer can be used for better results.

The liquid displacement method by using water or alcohol gives a density slightly less than true density of the powder since these liquids cannot enter into the smallest void space. This results in possible change in the true density values.

(ii) Gas displacement method: A weighted amount of the powder is introduced into the sample tube and already adsorbed gases are removed by degassing procedure. Helium gas which is not adsorbed by the powder is introduced. The pressure difference before and after the introduction of helium gas is obtained from a manometer. By applying gas laws, volume of helium surrounding the particles and penetrating into the small cracks and pores is calculated. The difference between the volume of helium filling the empty apparatus and the volume of helium filling in the presence of the powder gives the true volume of the powder. The true density can then be calculated. This method gives the closest value to true density as the helium can enter into all void spaces including pores and cracks.

Granular density (ρ_g)

It is determined by the method similar to liquid displacement method but mercury is employed as displacement liquid. The liquid mercury will not enter into the internal pores of the particles. Thus the granule volume represents the volume of the particles and intraparticle spaces. Intraparticulate volume may be open and closed. Open intraparticulate space is the space within a single particle that is open to the external environment whereas the closed intraparticulate space is the space within a single particle that is closed to the external environment.

Granular density $= \frac{\text{mass of the granular powder}}{\text{granule volume}}$

High compression density

In this method, the powder is highly compressed under a pressure of 100,000 lb/sq. inch into tablets. The ratio of the weight and its volume (obtained from tablet dimensions) gives the high compression density. These values are closer to true density.

Porosity of powders (ε)

Porosity is defined as the ratio of the void volume to the bulk volume of a powder packing

$$\varepsilon = \frac{\text{bulk volume} - \text{true volume}}{\text{bulk volume}}$$

$$= \frac{V_b - V_t}{V_b} = 1 - \frac{V_t}{V_b}$$

Porosity is also given as

$$\varepsilon = 1 - \frac{\text{weight/true density}}{\text{weight/bulk density}}$$

$$= 1 - \frac{\text{bulk density}}{\text{true density}}$$

or $$\frac{\text{true density} - \text{bulk density}}{\text{true density}}$$

The porosity calculated by using the true density value obtained from the gas adsorption method gives total porosity ($\varepsilon_{\text{total}}$) since the void space determined takes into account the intraparticle space and pores and cracks within the particles. (Fig. 4.14)

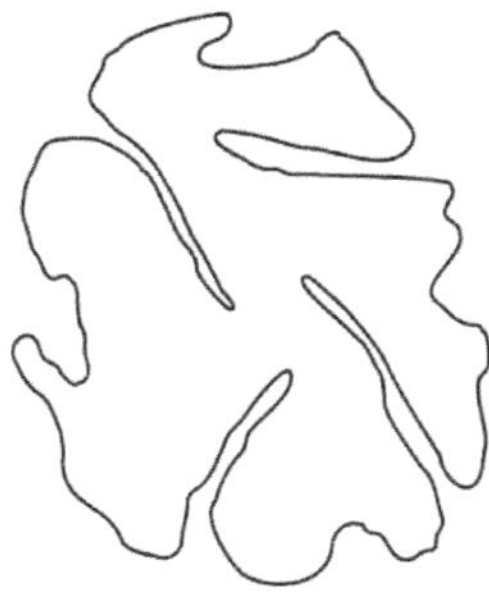

Fig. 4.14 Pores and Crevices in a Granule particle

$$\varepsilon_{\text{total}} = 1 - \frac{\text{bulk density}}{\text{true density}}$$

similarly

$$\varepsilon_{\text{interspace}} = 1 - \frac{\text{bulk density}}{\text{granule density}}$$

and $$\varepsilon_{\text{intraparticle}} = 1 - \frac{\text{granule density}}{\text{true density}}$$

Porosity is usually expressed as percent i.e, $\varepsilon \times 100$

Bulkiness

The reciprocal of bulk density is called bulk or bulkiness. It increases with a decrease in particle size. In a mixture of different sized particles, the bulkiness gets reduced since the smaller particles sift between the bigger particles. It is an important factor to be considered in the selection of suitable capsule size for a given dose of drug powder. It also serves as a guideline in choosing the containers for packaging. For example, light magnesium carbonate and light magnesium oxide may need a bigger container than that of the heavy magnesium carbonate and heavy magnesium oxide.

Packing arrangements of powder beds and heaps

A bed or a heap of powder contains a number of particles each in contact with its neighbors. Theoretically two types of packaging is possible. They are close packing or *rhombohedral packing* and open packing or *cubical packing* (Fig. 4.15).

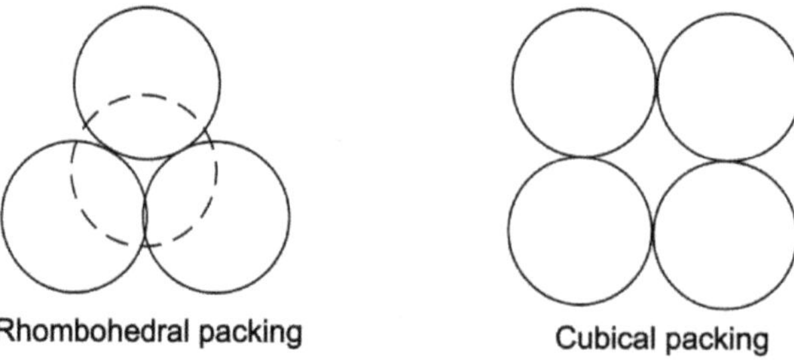

Fig. 4.15 Power Packing

The fraction of powder bed occupied by free space is called porosity. If the powder consists of isodiametric particles (spherical particles) and if the packing is open type the theoretical porosity is 48% and for close packing, it is 26%. But in practical situation, only a mixture of these two types of packing is possible and the porosity is around 30% or above. However, if the powder consists of different sized particles, the porosity may go below the theoretical minimum of 26%. This is because the smaller particles fill up the void spaces between the larger particles. On the other hand, if powder contains floccules or aggregates which lead to formation of bridges and arches in the packing, the porosity may go above the theoretical maximum of 48%.

Crystalline materials compressed into a hard core under a force of 100,000 lb/sq. inch can have porosities less than 1%.

If a powder is placed in a mechanical tapping device (Fig. 4.16) and tapped with the help of a rotating cam operated by a motor at a desired constant speed, there occurs a change in volume due to reduction in void space as more and more packing of particles occurs (i.e packing down). If the particles of the powder are spherical and monosize, the particles will take less time for packing down to a constant volume under the given conditions. Powders composed of non-isodiametric particles take much longer time to pack down to a constant volume.

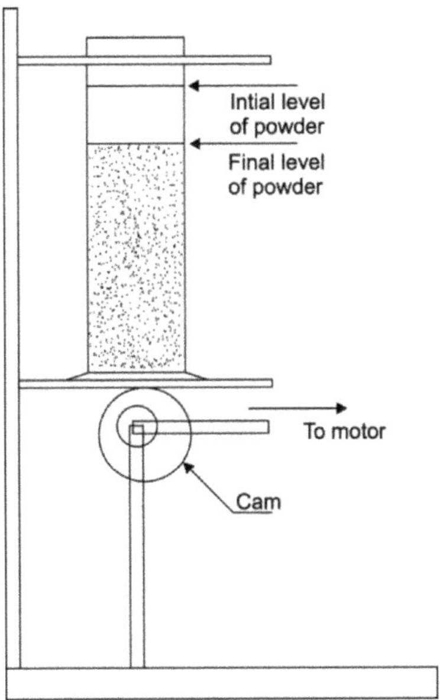

Fig. 4.16 Mechanical Tapping device

It is obvious that tablet granules (i.e granules for tableting) which are mostly both monosize and spherical will pack down rapidly. It helps to ensure uniform filling of the die to get constant weight tablets. That is why granulation is undertaken before compression of the drug powder into tablets.

Flow properties of powders and granules

A bulk powder is somewhat analogous to a non-Newtonian liquid as it exhibits plastic flow and sometimes dilatancy. In a powder, the flow of particles are influenced by attractive forces to varying degrees. Accordingly, the particles may be free flowing or sticky (cohesive). The various factors which decide the flow properties are particle size, shape, porosity, density and surface texture. The factors affecting flow properties may be called collectively as cohesive which is due to

1. surface forces between particles like *van der Waals* forces, surface tension, and electrostatic forces. These forces may cause the particles to adhere to the container.
2. inter particulate friction if the surface are rough and pitted.
3. interlocking of powder particles causing `bridging" and `arching'. For many powders these factors are difficult to be overcome by gravitational forces. Such powders are called sticky or cohesive.

The cohesion may be quantified as follows by using *Jenike cell* (Fig. 5.17)

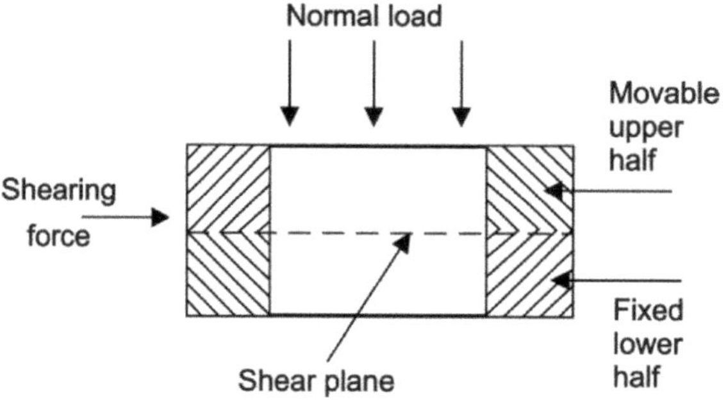

Fig. 4.17 Jenike cell

The powder is packed carefully into the two equal segments of a cell and a lid is placed on the top segment. A load is placed on the lid. The force required to just shear (that is the force just required to make the upper half to move) is found out by using a gauge. The experiment is repeated under different weights. The results are summarized as follows.

S.No.	Weight	Force required to shear
1	W_1	-
2	W_2	-
3	W_3	-
n	W_n	-

The values are plotted as follows shown in Fig. 4.18.

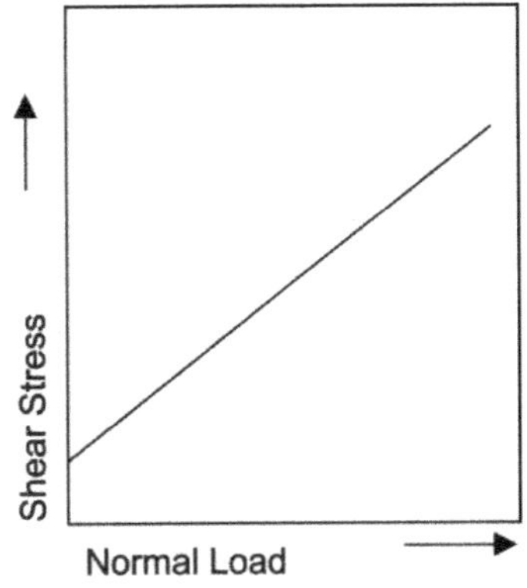

Fig. 4.18

The straight line obtained is extrapolated to meet the y-axis. The intercept point c which is the stress required to shear the bed under zero load is the actual cohesion force that exists between the particles of the powder. A highly cohesive powder tends to pack on storage and flow with difficulty and hence causes blocking of pipes and orifices. The cohesion is influenced by the following factors.

(a) Average particle size: Cohesion is a surface effect. Hence fine powders are more cohesive than coarse ones. Below 10 microns in size, the particles of most powders are extremely cohesive.

(b) Particle density: Dense substances are less cohesive than lighter ones.

(c) Nature of the surface: The surface of any particle is associated with surface free energy which is reduced by adsorption of gases and water vapour. In the absence of adsorption, there will be enormous cohesion. However. A continuous film of moisture also increases cohesion to a great extent.

Assessment of flow properties of powders

Flow property of a powder is usually assessed by determining angle of repose of the powders. For this, the powder is allowed to fall through an orifice from certain height, to form a conical heap of powder on a horizontal surface. The particle will slip and roll over each other when the heap is formed until the gravitational forces just balance the interparticular forces. The slanting side of the heap forms an angle with the horizontal surface which is known as angle of repose. The angle of repose is high if the cohesive and other forces are high. The angle of repose between 35 and 45 indicates the powder does not have satisfactory flow property. When the angle of repose is around 25 it indicates very good flow property. Flow property of powders play an important role during tablet manufacture and during capsule filling.

The angle of repose is measured as follows:

(i) The powder is allowed to fall over a paper placed on a horizontal surface through a funnel or an orifice kept at a certain convenient height (Fig. 4.19) or

(ii) cylindrical tube open at both the ends is placed on a paper on a horizontal surface so that one of the two open ends (i.e. the lower end) is closed on the surface of the paper. The powder is then, poured into the cylinder and the tube is gradually withdrawn without any shaking movements allowing the powder to form a heap on the horizontal surface. (Fig. 4.19)

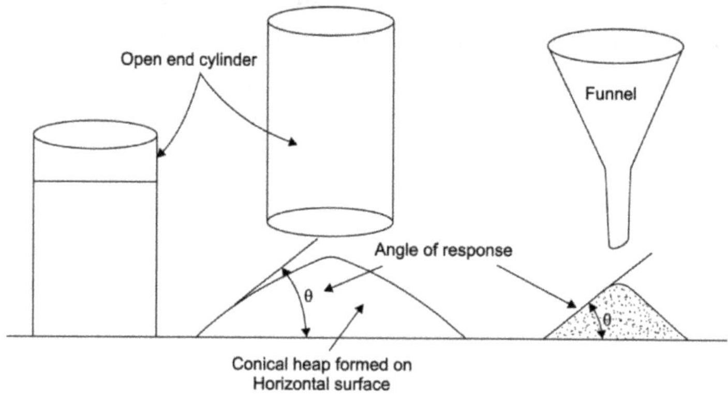

Fig. 4.19 Measurement of Angle of Repose

The height of the heap formed is measured by a suitable method and then the circumference of the base of the heap is drawn on the paper with the help of a pencil. The radius of the circle obtained, after removing the powder, is measured. The angle of repose is then given as

$$tan\ \theta = \frac{h}{r}$$

where θ = angle of repose

h = height of the heap

r = radius of the base of the heap (cone shaped heap)

The disadvantage of the funnel method is that it is suitable for free flowing powder only and it does not give reproducible results. The height through which the funnel should be raised to form heap is also critical and the force of fall of the powder through the funnel tube may compress the powder reducing the height of the powder. These difficulties may be overcome in the open ended cylindrical tube method.

In a dynamic method, a cylinder containing half filled powder is rotated slowly on a plane about its horizontal axis till the powder begins to cascade. The angle between horizontal plane and plane of the powder is the angle of repose. In yet an another dynamic method, the powder is taken fully in a rectangular box and the box is slowly lifted till the powder slides down. The angle between the horizontal surface and basal plane of the cylinder is the angle of repose.

Flow rates: Granular powders (have little cohesiveness because of symmetry of particles) show better flow rate than fine powders. As the proportion of fines increases, the flow rate of granules are decreased (above 40% fine, flow rate is suddenly decreased to low values)

Flow rate can be asserted by the following methods 1. The concerned material is allowed to fall through an orifice situated at the bottom of a cylinder. 2. By finding out compressibility index (I)

$$I = \left(1 - \frac{V}{V_o}\right) \times 100$$

where V = volume occupied by a sample of the powder after being tapped

by a standardized tapping procedure.

V_o volume before tapping.

For a powder with good flow property and flow rate, the value is below 15% and the values above 25% indicate poor flow property and the values between 15% and 25% indicate moderate flow property.

Improving the flow properties of powders

(a) If the powders contain a large proportion of fines, they may be removed by sieving or adsorbed over larger particles.
(b) If the cohesion is due to moisture present, the powder may be dried.
(c) By increasing the average size of the particle, the flow may be improved. Finer powders show cohesion. Granulation may be undertaken to increase the size and the flow property. In tablet technology, fine powder of the drugs and additives are converted to granules by dry granulation or by wet granulation techniques. Such a technique of conversion into granules is used even for nutritional foods and detergents.
(d) Presence of a small proportion of fine powder may improve the flow property due to the filling up of small crevices and pits present in coarse powders. In the absence of fine powder, a little amount of fine powder may be added.
(e) By producing isodiametric and symmetric particles like monosized spheres, the flow property can be increased. Such a requirement is met with spray dried products.
(f) Required particle size powders may be produced by suitable crystallisation or precipitation.
(g) By using additives like lubricants and glidants, the flow property may be increased. This is adopted to improve the flow property of granules in tablet technology.

Powders with improved flow properties are very essential in tablet technology wherein granules have to flow uniformly from the hopper to the die to produce tablets having uniform weights. In capsule technology also, uniform filling of capsules is assured only with free flowing powders. In cosmetic technology flow of powders such as face powders, tooth powders, dusting powders out of sifter top containers should be smooth enough.

The free-flowing powders are characterized by dustibility. Dustibility refers to the opposite of stickiness. The dustibility of Lycopodium (pollen grains) is arbitrarily taken as 100% . Talcum powder has a value of 57%, potato starch 27%, and fine charcoal 23%. Finely powdered calomel has a relative dustibility of 0.7%, these values have some relation to the uniform spreading of dusting powders (antibiotic dusting powders such as Novobiocin dusting powder) when applied to skin.

5. KINETICS

Introduction

A drug (or in its dosage form) may decompose or degrade or deteriorate under various conditions and because of various factors. In order to assure the therapeutic efficacy for the drug, it must be intact without decomposition. As the decomposition cannot be prevented completely, there is a need to assure a required concentration of the drug to elicit its pharmacologic actions. Therefore, the manufacturing chemist or dispensing pharmacist must be aware of those factors to assure maximum efficacy for the drug product.

The decomposition by chemical reaction may occur at different rates or speeds in a single reactant or between different reactants. The student must understand the reactant is the chemical entity in question and he is expected to know the order of chemical reactions or kinetics of reactions, methods of determining the order of reactions, the factors influencing the chemical reactions, and the methods to prevent such reactions to extend the life of the pharmaceutical products for patient's consumption at a later date.

Chemical kinetics

Chemical kinetics concerns with the study of rates of chemical reactions. A number of principles and related rate processes involved in the study of chemical kinetics are of immense help in the proper formulation and stabilization of pharmaceutical products.

Instability in formulations is mainly due to decomposition. The speed of decomposition follows the rate process. Dissolution as well as diffusion from solid dosage forms follows rate processes. The rate processes are also applicable to the study of absorption, distribution and elimination of drugs.

For a manufacturer, the principles of kinetics are of immense help in the performance of stability studies. Accelerated stability studies are undertaken to predict the stability of a product within a short period of time i.e., in determining the shelf-life of a product.

Thus, the principles studied under chemical kinetics provide a considerable advantage in the development of stable dosage forms. The manufacturer also gains considerable economic advantage in marketing a new product after formulation because of this approach. It is also possible to select the best formulation which will be stable for a long time from among a series of formulations.

Molecularity

A reaction may occur through several steps and each step is called an elementary step. Each elementary reaction has a stoichiometry giving the number of molecules taking part in the step. Since the order of an elementary reaction gives the number of molecules coming together to react in the step, it is referred to as molecularity of the elementary reaction. Simply, *molecularity* is the number of molecules, atoms, or ions reacting in an elementary reaction. Order (of a reaction) and molecularity are ordinarily identical only for elementary reactions. Bimolecular reactions may or may not be second order reaction.

The reaction, $Br_2 \rightarrow 2Br$ is unimolecular process, since a single bromine molecule decomposes to yield two bromine atoms.

The reaction, $H_2 + I_2 \rightarrow 2HI$ is a bimolecular process, since one hydrogen molecule and one iodine molecule (therefore two molecules) combine to yield hydrogen iodide.

Consider the experimentally determined *second order* reaction, $2NO + O_2 \rightarrow 2NO_2$. (The 2 in 2NO is the stochiometric coefficient). In this reaction, though three molecules (two NO molecules and one O_2 molecule) are involved, it is *not termolecular* process (the process in which three molecules collide together simultaneously to react is termed *termolecular*), because in the formation of two NO_2 molecules, the mechanism is postulated to consist of two elementary steps, each being bimolecular.

$$2NO \rightarrow N_2O_2 \quad \text{and } N_2O_2 + O_2 \rightarrow 2NO_2$$

Order of Reaction

The rate of a reaction refers to a change in concentration of the reactant with time. The order of a reaction refers to the way or manner in which the rate of the reaction changes with concentration of the reactants. It expresses the experimentally determined dependence of the reaction rate upon the concentration of the reactants.

First order reaction

When the rate of reaction is proportional to the first power of the concentration of a single reactant, the reaction is said to be first order with respect to the single reactant.

In this order of reaction, a single reactant decomposes directly into one or more products and may be represented as follows

$$A \longrightarrow \text{products}$$

$$\frac{d\,[A]}{dt} \qquad \dots (1)$$

Then, the rate of reaction is directly proportional to the concentration of the reacting substance $[A]$. Expressing this mathematically at any time t after replacing $[A]$ by C

The equation (1) can be written as

$$-\frac{dC}{dt} = kC^n \qquad \dots (2)$$

or, $-\frac{dC}{dt} = kC^1$ for first order reaction

Separating the variables, we can write equation (2) as

$$-\frac{dC}{dt} = k\,dt \qquad \dots (3)$$

in which C is the concentration of reactant remaining unreacted (or undecomposed) at time t, and k is the first order rate constant.

Integrating the equation (3) between the limits when $C = C_0$ (initial concentration) at $t = 0$ and $C = C$ at $t = t$

$$-\int_{C_0}^{C} \frac{dC}{C} = k \int_{0}^{t} dt$$

$$-(\ln C - \ln C_0) = k\,(t - 0)$$

$$-\ln C + \ln C_0 = kt$$

Multiplying both sides by minus (–) we obtain

$$\ln C - \ln C_0 = -kt$$

$$\text{or, } \ln C = \ln C_0 - kt \qquad \text{... (4)}$$

Converting the natural logarithm into common logarithm, we can write, equation (4) as

$$2.303\ \log C = 2.303\ \log C_0 - kt$$

Dividing both sides of equation with the factor 2.303 yields,

$$\log C = \log C_0 - \frac{kt}{2.303} \qquad \text{... (5)}$$

This equation describes the first order kinetics as a function of logarithm of concentration, time and reaction rate constant.

The value of k for the reaction is calculated from the slope obtained by plotting $\ln C$ or $\log C$ against time, t, using the linear form of equation (4) or (5). The slope is equal to $-k$ if equation (4) is used for plotting and it is $-k/2.303$ if equation (5) is used for plotting. The rate constant, k, for first order reaction has units of *reciprocal time (time^{-1})*

The straight line (Fig. 5.1-B) produced by plotting $\ln C$ or $\log C$ against t is an identifying characteristic of first order reaction in which the rate of reaction is proportional to the concentration of a single reactant.

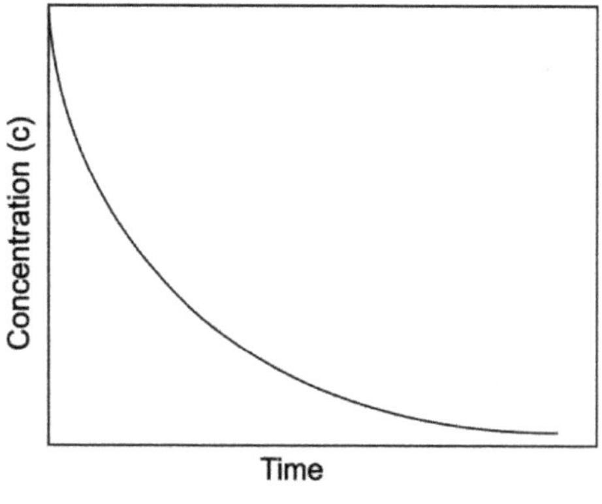

Fig. 5.1A

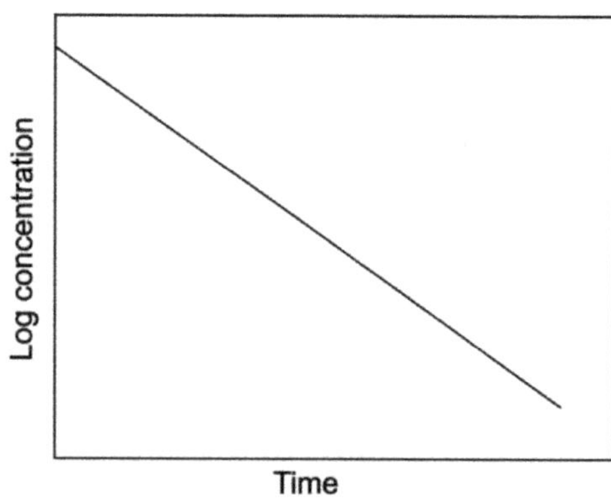

Fig. 5.1B

The equation (5) can be rearranged to obtain

$$k = \frac{2.303}{t} \log \frac{C_0}{C} \qquad \text{... (6)}$$

A modification of this equation is that, C_0, the initial concentration is replaced by a and C by $(a - x)$, the concentration remaining unreacted and x, is the concentration reacted at time t. It is given as

$$k = \frac{2.303}{t} \log \frac{a}{a - x} \qquad \text{... (7)}$$

Sometimes, C_0 either is not known or is not a suitable reference concentration. In such cases, the equation (3) may be integrated between the limits $C = C_1$ at $t = t_1$ and $C = C_2$ at $t = t_2$

$$-\int_{C_1}^{C_2} \frac{dC}{C} = -k \int_{t_1}^{t_2} dt$$

$$-(\ln C_2 - \ln C_1) = k\,(t_2 - t_1)$$

$$-\ln C_2 + \ln C_1 = k\,(t_2 - t_1)$$

$$k = \frac{\ln C_1 - \ln C_2}{t_2 - t_1} \qquad \text{... (8)}$$

$$\text{or,}\quad k = \frac{\ln C_1 - \ln C_2}{t_2 - t_1} \qquad \text{... (9)}$$

The equation (7) may be written in logarithmic form as

$$k = \frac{2.303}{t_2 - t_1} \log \frac{C_1}{C_2} \qquad \text{... (10)}$$

The concentration terms in the first order kinetics express the fact that the concentration decreases exponentially with time. This can be understood by referring to a graph (Fig. 5.1A) obtained by plotting concentration against time. Equation of first order kinetics can, then, be written in an exponential form as follows

$$\ln C = \ln C_0 - kt$$

$$\ln \frac{C}{C_0} = -kt$$

Taking inverse logarithms on both sides of equation, we can write

$$\frac{C}{C_0} = e^{-kt}$$

The above equation can be given as

$$C = C_0 \,.\, e^{-kt} \qquad \text{... (11)}$$

$$\text{Or} \quad C_0 = C \,.\, e^{kt} \qquad \text{... (12)}$$

Some examples of first order reaction are

(a) Inversion of cane sugar

In dilute solutions of sucrose, the active mass of water does not change appreciably. The rate of chemical reaction depends upon concentration of sucrose only. In the stoichiometric equation, only one molecule of sucrose is involved hence it is considered to follow first order kinetics.

(b) Hydrolysis of methyl acetate

$$CH_3COOCH_3 + H_2O \rightleftharpoons CH_3COOH + CH_3OH$$

In this water is taken in larger quantity and hence active mass of water is not changed appreciably. Although two molecules (in the stoichiometric equation) react in the equation, only one molecule is considered to be involved in the reaction with change in concentration and therefore it is called pseudo first order kinetic reaction.

(c) Decomposition of procaine hydrochloride in ammonium hydroxide-hydrochloric acid buffer, pH 9.7, at 50°C. It follows pseudo first order kinetic.

(d) Decomposition of hydrogen peroxide in aqueous solution in the presence of finely divided platinum

$$H_2O_2 \longrightarrow H_2O + O$$

(e) Radioactive disintegration

(f) Decomposition of nitrogen peroxide

$$N_2O_5 \longrightarrow 2NO_2 + (O)$$

Half-life of reactants

By observing the figure (5.1A), one can understand that theoretically first order reaction takes infinite period of time for the completion of the reaction (i.e., for all the reactant to undergo reaction). Hence, a statement of time needed for complete decomposition would be meaningless. Actually, the rate subsides ordinarily in a finite period of time at which the reaction may be considered to be almost complete. Hence it is quite satisfactory to calculate what is called half-life rather than the time required for a substance to decompose completely.

Half-life of a reactant may be indicated by symbols such as $t_{1/2}$, or $t_{50\%}$. It is defined as the time required for the initial concentration of a reactant to get reduced to half its initial value in a reaction. Simply, it is the time required for the reactant to reach 50% concentration of its initial value because of decomposition. It may also be defined as the time required for half of the reactant to undergo reaction. Suppose a product contained an initial concentration of 10 mg / 5 ml of a drug, then the time required for half of the drug to get decomposed would be the half-life i.e. the time required for the product to get reduced to 5 mg / 5 ml of the drug would be the half-life of the product. If a first order reaction is followed through 10 half-lives, less than 0.1% of initial concentration of a reactant will remain unreacted. However, in practice, it is often enough to follow through two or three half-life periods.

The half-life may be obtained as follows for the first order reaction.

$$t = \frac{2.303}{k} \log \frac{C_0}{C}$$

$$t_{1/2} = \frac{2.303}{k} \log \frac{C_0}{1/2\ C_0}$$

$$= \frac{2.303}{k} \log 2$$

$$t_{1/2} = \frac{0.693}{k} \qquad \text{... (13)}$$

In pharmaceutical field, the time for the drug to decompose by 10% is an important value to know. It is also important to note that $t_{1/2}$ or $t_{50\%}$ does not depend on concentration. That is, it takes the same time for the concentration of the drug to go from 0.5 mole to 0.25 mole as it would take to go from 0.01 mole to 0.005 mole.

1. *The catalytic decomposition of hydrogen peroxide may be followed by measuring the volume of oxygen liberated in a gas burette. When such a study was undertaken it was found that the concentration of hydrogen peroxide remaining after 45 minutes was 16.70 i.e. the volume of gas in ml evolved from hydrogen peroxide whose concentration of oxygen in ml was initially 57.90. Calculate the rate constant k using first order rate equation. How much of hydrogen peroxide remained after 10 minutes ?*

$$k = \frac{2.303}{t} \log \frac{c_o}{c}$$

Substituting the values, $k = \frac{2.303}{45} \log \frac{57.90}{16.70}$

$$= \mathbf{0.0276\ min^{-1}}$$

The amount of hydrogen peroxide remained after 10 minutes would be

$$\text{Log } c = \log c_o - \frac{kt}{2.303}$$

Substituting the value

$$\log c = \log 57.90 - \frac{0.0276 \times 10}{2.303}$$

$$\log c = 1.7627 - 0.1198 = 1.6429$$

The anti-log of 1.6429 is 42.94 i.e., c =43.94

The amount of hydrogen peroxide remaining after 10 minutes would be ***43.94 ml***

2. *The first order rate constant k for the acid catalyzed hydrolysis of benzocaine is* $14.0 \times 10^{-6}\ sec^{-1}$*. Calculate half-life of the drug.*

Half-life for first order reaction is $\frac{0.693}{k}$

Substituting the values, half-life is $= \frac{0.693}{140 \times 10^{-6}}$ *=4960 seconds*

or ***82.5 minutes***

3. *Menadione (vit K_2) is degraded by exposure to light, which is called photodegradation or photolysis. The rate constant of decomposition k is 4.863 × 10^{-3} min^{-1}. Compute the half life.*

Half-life for first order reaction is $\frac{\mathbf{0.693}}{\boldsymbol{k}}$

Substituting the values, half-life is = $\frac{\mathbf{0.693}}{\mathbf{4.863 \times 10^{-3}}}$

=142.5 min or 2 hr 22 min

4. *A drug product contains 500 mg/ml of a drug in solution. If the decomposition follows first order kinetics, what will be the amount left after 2 half-life periods and after 4 half-life periods?*

*Answer: The initial concentration is 400 mg/ml. After first half-life period, the amount left unreacted will be 400/2 = 200 mg/ml. After second half-life period, the amount left will be 200/2 =**100 mg/ml**. After 4 half-life periods the amount remaining will be **25 mg/ml.***

Second order reaction

A second order reaction refers to a reaction in which the experimentally determined rate of reaction is proportional either to second power of the concentration of a single reactant or to the first power of the concentrations of two reactants.

If two reactants A and B react at a rate proportional to the concentration of each i.e., $[A]$ and $[B]$, we can write

$$-\frac{d\,[A]}{dt} = -\frac{d\,[B]}{dt} = k\,[A][B]$$

If a and b represent the initial concentrations of A and B respectively and x is the amount of each of A and B reacting in time t, the reaction rate $\frac{dx}{dt}$ is given as

$$\frac{dx}{dt} = k\,(a - x)(b - x) \qquad \text{... (14)}$$

Where $(a - x)$ and $(b - x)$ represent the concentration of A and B remaining unreacted at time t.

For a simple case, if the initial concentration of A and B are equal (i.e., $a = b$) the above equation (14) can be written as

$$\frac{dx}{dt} = k\,(a - x)^2 \qquad \text{... (15)}$$

On integration between the limits $x = 0$ at t = 0 and $x = x$ at $t = t$.

$$\int_0^x \frac{dx}{(a - x)^2} = k \int_0^t dt$$

$$\left(\frac{1}{a - x}\right) - \left(\frac{1}{a - 0}\right) = kt$$

$$\frac{x}{a\,(a - x)} = kt \qquad \text{... (16)}$$

Or $$\frac{1}{a} \cdot \frac{x}{(a - x)} = kt$$

Or $$\frac{1}{at} \cdot \frac{x}{(a - x)} = k \qquad \text{... (17)}$$

If the initial concentrations of A and B are not equal (i.e., $a \neq b$), integration of the equation (14) yields.

$$\frac{2.303}{(a - b)} \log \frac{b\,(a - x)}{a\,(b - x)} = kt \qquad \text{... (17a)}$$

If $x/a\,(a - x)$ is plotted against t with reference to equation (16), it will yield a straight line. The slope of the line gives the value of k.

If the initial concentrations of A and B are not equal, the equation (17a) is used for plotting. That is, if log $b\ (a - x)/\ a\ (b - x)$ is plotted against t, it will yield a straight line. Then the slope of the line is given by $(a - b)\ k\ /\ 2.303$

The rate constant k for a *second order reaction has units of liter mole^{-1} sec^{-1}*

The half-life for a second order reaction is obtained as follows

Consider the equation (17)

$$k = \frac{1}{at}\frac{x}{a - x}$$

At $t = t_{1/2}, x = \frac{1}{2}a$

Substituting these values in the equation

$$k = \frac{1}{at_{1/2}}\frac{1/2a}{a - 1/2a}$$

$$k = \frac{1}{at_{1/2}}\frac{\frac{1}{2}a}{1/2a}$$

$$k = \frac{1}{at_{1/2}}$$

On rearrangement,

$$t_{1/2} = \frac{1}{ak} \text{ or } t_{1/2} \propto \frac{1}{a} \qquad \text{... (18)}$$

In second order reactions $t_{1/2}$ is significant only when a single reactant or when two reactants of same initial concentrations are involved.

The most common rate processes encountered in the consideration of drug stability are the first and second order reactions. When a reaction happens to be of higher order, it is always convenient to adjust the experimental conditions in such a way that except the concentration of one reactant, all the other concentrations of reactants are made to remain constant throughout the experiment. For example, the saponification of an ester by hydroxide (NaOH or KOH) is second order reaction. This second order reaction can be made to follow first order kinetics provided the hydroxide is taken in great excess or the hydroxide ion is maintained constant by using a buffer system. The actual rate constant k is then obtained by dividing the experimentally determined apparent first order rate constant by the concentration of hydroxide ion maintained constant throughout the experiment. Thus, a *pseudo* or *apparent* first order reaction can be defined as a second order reaction or bimolecular reaction that is made to behave like a first order reaction. In such a reaction, the rate is determined by one of the reactants even though two reactants are present since the second reactant does not show significant changes in concentration. Hydrolysis of an ester in presence of large excess of water is an example of *pseudo* first order reaction whereas the hydrolysis of an ester by using alkali is the second order reaction.

Examples of second order reactions are

(a) Decomposition of ozone into oxygen

$$2O_3 \longrightarrow 3O_2$$

(b) Conversion of benzaldehyde to benzoin

$$2C_6H_5CHO \longrightarrow 2C_6H_5CH\,(OH)\,COC_6H_5$$

(c) Hydrolysis of an ester by an alkali

$$CH_3COOC_2H_5 + NaOH \rightleftharpoons CH_3COONa + C_2H_5OH$$

Ethyl acetate is mixed with an equal quantity of sodium hydroxide solution and the reaction mixture is kept at a constant temperature. In the stoichiometric equation two species of molecules are involved in the reaction and both undergo appreciable change in their concentration and hence, it is called second order kinetic reaction.

(d) Decomposition of chlorbutol in sodium hydroxide solution at 25°C follows second order kinetic reaction.

(e) Thermal decomposition of acetaldehyde follows second order reaction.

$$2CH_3CHO \longrightarrow 2CH_4 + 2CO$$

5. *Saponification of an ester at a temperature of 25°C with sodium hydroxide was investigated the initial concentration of both the ester and alkali in the mixture was 0.005 M. The change in concentration of alkali during 30 minutes was 0,0028 mole/liter. Compute the rate constant and half-life.*

Because of both the ester and alkali take part in the reaction and are of equal concentrations, it is second order reaction. In such a reaction the decrease in concentration in one of the reactants is equal to the decrease in concentration of the other reactant. Therefore, the change in concentration (of 0.0028) in alkali is also the change in concentration of the ester and it gives the value of x which indicates the amount reacted and $(\mathbf{a}-\mathbf{x})$ *indicates the remaining concentration at the end of 30 minutes. Therefore, a = 0.005 and* $(\mathbf{a}-\mathbf{x})$ *= 0.005 – 0.0028 = 0.0022. The second order rate constant equation is*

$$\boldsymbol{k} = \frac{1}{at}\left(\frac{x}{a-x}\right)$$

Substituting the values in the above second order reaction formula,

$$\boldsymbol{k} = \frac{1}{0.005 \times 30}\left(\frac{0.0028}{0.0022}\right)$$

$$k = \frac{0.0028}{0.00033} = 8.48 \text{ liter mole}^{-1}\text{min}^{-1}$$

Half-life for second order reaction is given by $t_{1/2} = \frac{1}{ak}$

Substituting the values, $\frac{1}{0.005 \times 8.48}$ $=$ **235 minutes**

Or **3.93 hours**

6. *The initial concentration of both ethyl acetate in the mixture was 0.01mole/liter. the rate constant for the reaction was found to be 4.62 liters. mole.*$^{-1}$ *min.*$^{-1}$ *Compute the half-life of the ester.*

Half-life for second order reaction is given by $t_{1/2} = \frac{1}{ak}$

Substituting the values in the equation, $t_{1/2} = \frac{1}{0.01 \times 4.62}$

= **21.64 minutes**

Third order reaction

A third order reaction refers to a reaction in which the experimentally determined reaction rate is proportional to

1. the first power concentration of each of the three reactants or
2. the first power concentration of one of the two reactants and to the second power of the second reactant or
3. the third power of the concentration of a single reactant.

It may be represented as

$$A + B + C \longrightarrow \text{products or}$$

$$2A + B \longrightarrow \text{products or}$$

$$A + 2B \longrightarrow \text{products or}$$

$$3A \longrightarrow \text{products}$$

For the reaction

$$A + B + C \longrightarrow \text{products, the rate low is:}$$

$$-\frac{d[A]}{dt} = \frac{d[B]}{dt} = k\,[A][B][C]$$

If a, b and c represent the concentrations of A, B and C respectively and when $a = b = c$,

$$\frac{dx}{dt} = k\,(a - x)^3$$

On integration, the equation will yield

$$k = \frac{1}{2t}\left[\frac{1}{(a - x)^2} - \frac{1}{a^2}\right] \quad \text{... (19)}$$

When t= $t_{1/2}, x = 0.5a$ or $1/2a$ and on substitution in equation (19)

$$t_{1/2} = \frac{1}{a^2} \times \frac{1.5}{k} \text{ and } t_{1/2} \propto \frac{1}{a^2} \quad \text{... (20)}$$

Examples of third order reactions are

(a) Formation of nitrogen peroxide

$$O_3 + 2NO \longrightarrow 2NO_2$$

(b) Reduction of ferric chloride by stannous chloride

$$2FeCl_3 + SnCl_2 \longrightarrow 2FeCl_2 + SnCl_4$$

Zero order reactions

In certain reactions, the rate of chemical reaction is independent of the concentration of the reactant molecules and is known as zero order reaction. It is mathematically expressed as

$$-\frac{d[A]}{dt} = k_0 \,.\, [A]^0 \quad \text{... (21)}$$

Writing C^0 for $[A]^0$, the equation (21) becomes

$$-\frac{dc}{dt} = k_0 C^0 \quad \text{... (22)}$$

Where k_0 = rate constant for zero order reaction. Since $C^0 = 1$, the equation is written as

$$-\frac{dc}{dt} = k_0 \quad \text{... (23)}$$

The above equation shows that the rate of reaction in zero order kinetics is independent of concentration of the reactant but it proceeds at a fixed rate. The fixed rate is k, the rate constant. That is, the concentration decreases at a fixed rate irrespective of the initial concentration of the reactant. Thus, if a drug in a product degrades at the rate of 1.0 mg per day, the rate of degradation will be 1.0 mg / day irrespective of initial concentration of the drug in the product. Suppose the initial concentration of the drug in the product was 100 mg, then the drug would be completely degraded in 100 days.

The above equation (23) may be written as

$$-dC = k_0\, dt \qquad \text{... (24)}$$

Integrating the equation between the limits when $C = C_1$ at $t - t_1$ and $C - C_2$ at $t = t_2$, (where $C_1 > C_2$ and $t_1 > t_2$)

$$-\int_{C_1}^{C_2} dC = k_0 \int_{t_1}^{t_2} dt$$

$$-(C_2 - C_1) = k_0\,(t_2 - t_1)$$

Rearranging the above equation, we obtain

$$k_0 = -\left(\frac{C_2 - C_1}{t_2 - t_1}\right) = \frac{C_1 - C_2}{t_2 - t_1} \text{ or } \frac{C_2 - C_1}{t_1 - t_2} \qquad \text{... (25)}$$

The equation (24) may also be integrated between the limits $C = C_0$ at $t = 0$ and $C = C_t$ at $t = t$.

$$-\int_{C_0}^{C_t} dC = k_0 \int_{0}^{t} dt$$

$$-(C_t - C_0) = k_0\,(t - 0)$$

or,
$$C_0 - C_t = k_0 t \qquad \text{... (26)}$$

Or,
$$C_0 = C_t + k_0 t \qquad \text{... (27)}$$

Or,
$$C_t = C_0 - k_0 t \qquad \text{... (28)}$$

The equation indicates that concentration in a zero-order reaction at any time t is equal to the initial concentration minus the product of reaction rate constant and time.

(Sometimes, $(C_0 - C_t)$ is replaced by x, the concentration reacted in time t and the equation becomes $x = k\,t$)

In multi-sulfa product, the velocity of color fading is found to be constant and is independent of concentration of the colorant used. That is, color fading follows zero order kinetics. Then, the equation is given by

$$A_t = A_0 - k_0 t \quad \text{... (29)}$$

Where A_t = absorbance at $t = t$

A_0 = absorbance at $t = 0$

k_0 = zero order rate constant

Pseudo-order reactions

For some reactions, the rate of reaction may not depend on the concentration of one or more of the reactants over a wide range of concentrations. They may occur under the following conditions.

a) One or more of the reactants enters into the rate equation in great excess when compared to the others.

b) One of the reactants is a catalyst.

c) One or more of the reactants is constantly replenished during the course of reaction

For example, consider the following equation,

$$C_{12}H_{22}O_{11} + H_2O \rightarrow C_6H_{12}O_6 + C_6H_{12}O_6$$

(sucrose + water → glucose + fructose)

The reaction is known to be a second order according to the definition of second order reaction. For most reactions in aqueous solutions, the molar concentration of water (approximately 55.5 mole of water per liter) greatly exceeds the concentration of the solute, sucrose. This allows only the concentration of sucrose to be considered, and hence, the reaction is considered to be *an apparent (pseudo) first order reaction*

In some pharmaceutical preparations such as suspensions, degradation follows zero-order kinetics. In suspensions, the concentration of a drug in solution depends on the drug's equilibrium solubility. As the drug in solution decomposes, the drug in solid in suspended form will go into solution so that the concentration of drug in solution remains constant (i.e. the amount reacted is instantly replaced by dissolution of the drug). It is to be understood that the drug's concentration in solution remains constant despite its degradation with time because the solid drug acts as reservoir of drug.

The equation for the degradation of that drug in solution is the same for an ordinary solution of the drug with no reservoir of drug to replace that depleted or decomposed. That is, the degradation follows first order kinetics and is given by

$$-\frac{dC}{dt} = kC$$

where C is the concentration of drug remaining undecomposed at time `t' and k is known as the first order rate constant. When C is rendered constant (as in suspension), the above first order reaction becomes,

$$-\frac{dC}{dt} = k_0$$

where k_0 is rate constant for zero order reaction and the equation is *apparent or pseudo-zero order equation*. It should also be understood that once all the suspended particles have gone into solution, the reaction changes to first order kinetics.

Half-life of zero order

The half-life of a zero-order reaction can be obtained from the equation

$$C_t = C_0 - k_0 t$$

The half-life $(t_{1/2})$ is the time when C_t is equal to $\frac{1}{2}\,C_0$ Substituting these values in the above equation, we get

$$\frac{1}{2}\,C_0 = C_0 - k_0\,t_{1/2}$$

On rearranging, it gives

$$t_{1/2} = \frac{C_0 - \frac{1}{2}C_0}{k_0} = \frac{\frac{1}{2}C_0}{k_0} \qquad \text{... (30)}$$

$$t_{1/2} = \frac{C_0}{2k_0}$$

The initial concentration corresponding to C_0 is ordinarily written as `a' and hence $t_{1/2}$ can also be written as

$$t_{1/2} = \frac{a}{2k_0} \qquad \text{... (31)}$$

Examples of zero order reactions are

(a) Decomposition of hydrogen iodide at the surface of gold. At sufficiently higher pressure, the catalyst surface is covered by HI molecules and thus the concentration of the reactant remains constant throughout the reaction.

(b) In hydrogen iodide formation, the concentrations of hydrogen and iodine, have no effect on the reaction, but exposure to sunlight will induce the reaction spontaneously between hydrogen and iodine to yield hydrogen iodide. This photochemical reaction follows zero order kinetics.

(c) Decomposition of sparingly soluble drugs in aqueous solution follow zero order kinetics (the apparent zero order) since the amount of drug decomposed in the solution is replaced by the dissolution of some of the suspended drug and thus the concentration of the drug in the solution remains constant e.g. suspension of asprin.

(d) Color fading in multi-sulfa formulation.

6. *Absorption of a freshly prepared colored multi-sulphonamide product was measured in a photo-calorimeter at 500 nm and the absorption (at time zero) was found to be o.470 at 25°C. After at t = 60 hours, the absorption was found to be 0.270. As the color fading is independent of concentration, it follows zero order reaction. Calculate the (apparent) zero order rate constant k_o and the half life of the product.*

Rate constant for the (apparent) zero order reaction (in terms of absorbance) is

$$At = A_o - kt$$

$$\text{Then, } k = \frac{-A_t + A_o}{t}$$

Substituting the values in the above equation, $\mathbf{k} = \frac{-0.270+0.470}{60} = \frac{0.2}{60}$

$$k = 3.3 \times 10^{-3}$$

Half-life for zero order reaction is $t_{1/2} = \frac{a}{2k} = \frac{0.470}{0.0033} = \mathbf{142.42\ hours}$

or ***5.93 days or nearly 6 days***

7. *The apparent zero order rate constant in a suspension was reported to be 1.5 × 10^{-6} g/100 ml/sec. If the initial concentration is 400 ml/5 ml, calculate the shelf life of the product assuming that the product is satisfactory until the time at which it has decomposed to 90% of its original concentration or by 10% of its concentration.*

5 ml contains 400 mg, then, 100 ml contains (400×100/5) 8 g i.e., c_o = 8 g and the rate constant, $\mathbf{k_o}$ *is 1.5 × 10^{-6} g/100 ml/sec. Then, $t_{90\%}$ for zero order is given by*

$$t_{90\%} = \frac{0.10 \times c_o}{k_o}$$

Substituting the values in the equation,

$$t_{90\%} = \frac{0.10 \times 8}{1.5 \times 10^{-6}} = 533333 \text{ seconds or}$$

= ***370 days***

8. *Absorption of a multi-sulfa product was 0.470 at 500 nm at time zero. The order of reaction, k_o was found to be 0.00082 absorbance decrease per hour at 60°C signifying zero order kinetics. Compute the half-life for the product.*

$$t_{1/2} = \frac{a}{2k} \text{ or } \frac{1/2a}{k}$$

$$= \frac{0.470}{2 \times 0.00082} = \mathbf{286.6\ hours.}$$

Or **11.94 days**

Reactions of higher order

Tetramolecular and higher order reactions are very rare since chance of simultaneous collisions of more molecules at a time is not possible as per kinetic molecular theory.

Methods to determine the order of reaction

Substitution method

The most obvious method is the one in which the quantities a, x and t are determined experimentally and the values are substituted in the respective order of reaction. The equation that yields a constant value of k for a series of time intervals indicates the order of reaction.

Graphical method

This is a simple method. In this, instead of substituting the values in the respective equations of the order of reaction, the values are used to plot a graph.

If a straight line is obtained by plotting the concentration (a) against time (t), it indicates a zero-order reaction. If $\log(a - x)$ versus t yields a straight line, it is first order. For a second order a plot of $\frac{1}{(a-x)}$ versus t yields a straight line provided the initial concentration of the two reactants involved in the reaction are same. The reaction is of third order when a plot of $\frac{1}{(a-x)^2}$ versus t results in a straight line with all the three reactants at the same initial concentrations.

Half-life method

In general, the half-life ($t_{1/2}$) of a reaction in which the concentrations of all reactants are equal, the half-life, $(t_{1/2})$, is given by

$t_{1/2} \propto \frac{1}{a^{n-1}}$ where $n =$ order of the reaction.

Starting with two different initial concentrations a_1 and a_2 for the same reaction, the half-lives $(t_{1/2})_1$ and $(t_{1/2})_2$ are determined respectively. Then, the order of reaction,

$$n = \frac{\log (t_{1/2})_1 - \log (t_{1/2})_2}{\log a_2 - \log a_1} + 1$$

Where, $n =$ order of the reaction.

The half-lives can be determined by plotting a versus t at two different concentrations a_1 and a_2, Then, the half time at $\frac{1}{2}\, a_1$ and $\frac{1}{2}\, a_2$ are read from the graph. The values obtained are substituted in the above equation and n is arrived at and that gives the order of reaction.

If $(t_{1/2})_1 = (t_{1/2})_2$, it is first order reaction since in a first order $t_{1/2}$ is independent of concentration `a'. For a zero-order $t_{1/2}$ is proportional to the initial concentration$a$. For a second order in which $a = b$ (i.e. in which the concentration of the reactant A is equal to the concentration of the reactant B), $t_{1/2}$ is proportional to $\frac{1}{a}$ and for third order in which $a = b = c$, $t_{1/2}$ is proportional to $\frac{1}{a^2}$.

Complex Reactions

Reactions are not as simple as the stoichiometric equation would show. Hence it is not possible to express many reactions by simple zero, first, second or third-order.

Very often two or more reactions take place at the same time. Accordingly, they are called complex reactions. They may be

1. Reversible reaction (or opposing reactions)

$$A + B \rightleftharpoons C + D$$

2. Parallel or side reactions (or simultaneous reaction)

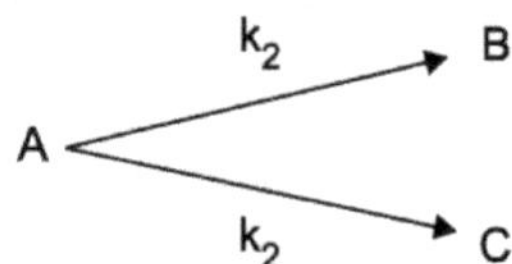

e.g., General acid base catalysed reactions.

3. Series or consecutive reactions.

$$A \underset{k_1}{\rightarrow} B \underset{k_2}{\rightarrow} C$$

e.g., Depletion of glucose in acid solution and degradation of hydrocortisone semisuccinate at 70°C over a narrow pH range.

Decomposition of chlorthiazide gives a final product which is produced by a series of consecutive first order kinetics.

Theoretically, all reactions are reversible. In most of the cases, the reverse reaction may be disregarded as it does not alter the concentration very much. If the reverse reaction cannot be ignored, the equilibrium constant must be taken into account in the evaluation of specific reaction rate constant.

For the kinetic study of chemical reactions in the case of consecutive reactions, the reaction which proceeds at a slower rate may be considered. If a number of steps are involved in a reaction, the slowest of the steps is the rate determining step for the overall reaction.

Parallel reactions are quite common particularly in organic compounds. In the kinetic study, the one which predominates over all the other is selected.

Experiments may show a reaction order which is non-integral or fractional for complex reactions. In spite of that, the order of reaction with respect to each reactant can be determined by controlling the concentrations of other reactants. In this way the integral reaction order with respect to each component can be arrived at.

Steady state approximation: Michaelis Menton Equation

The rate laws of a number of kinetic processes cannot be integrated exactly. It is better to postulate a reasonable reaction sequence and then the rate law may be derived.

The steady state approximation may be employed to derive the rate law. This may be illustrated by deriving the Michaelis Menton equation

Michaelis and Menton assumed the interaction between a drug (or substrate) D, with an enzyme E to yield product, P.

The sequence of reaction may be represented as follows

$$E + D \underset{k_2}{\overset{k_1}{\rightleftharpoons}} (E.D) \xrightarrow{k_a} P$$

Where $E.D$ is the (drug-enzyme) complex which ultimately yields the product`P'.

Then, the rate of product formation is given by

$$\frac{dp}{dt} = k_3\,[E.D] \qquad \text{... (32)}$$

Under steady state, the above equation (32) may be written as

$$\frac{dp}{dt} = k_3\,[E.D]_{SS} \qquad \text{... (33)}$$

$where,\ [E.D]_{SS} = \frac{DE_t}{k_m + D}$ (the derivation of this equation is not considered here)

Substituting for $[E.D]_{SS}$ into equation (33)

$$\frac{dp}{dt} = \frac{k_3 DE_t}{k_m + D} \qquad \text{... (34)}$$

Where k_m is Michaelis-Menton constant which is equal to $k_2 + k_1 / k_1$, and

E_t = total concentration of enzyme

When D is present in very large excess, all the enzyme E_t is present as $E.D$. In otherwords, all the enzyme is combined with the drug and reaction proceeds at maximum velocity i.e. $\left(\frac{dp}{dt}\right)_{max}$

Replacing $\left(\frac{dp}{dt}\right)_{max}$ by V and $k_3 E_t$ by V_m and since $[E.D]$ is equivalent to E_t, the equation (34) becomes

$$V = \frac{V_m D}{k_m + D} \qquad \text{... (35)}$$

The equation (35) may be inverted to obtain the linear form of equation which is known as Lineweaver-Bunk equation.

$$\frac{1}{V} = \frac{k_m}{V_m} \cdot \frac{1}{D} + \frac{1}{V_m} \qquad \text{... (36)}$$

A plot of $\frac{1}{V}$ versus $\frac{1}{D}$ gives a straight line with an intercept $\frac{1}{V_m}$ in the ordinate. The slope is k_m/V_m.

It is possible to calculate k_m, the Michaeles-Menton constant from the values of V_m and k_m/V_m

The kinetics of capacity limited of saturable processes can best be described by Michaeles-Menton equation.

Factors Influencing Reaction Rates

Many factors affect the rate of reaction ***other than concentration***. They are:

1. Temperature

In general, the rate of degradation increases with rise in temperature. Usually, it increases by a factor of between two and three-fold for every 10°C rise in temperature.

The influence of temperature on the reaction velocity k is given quantitatively by Arrhenius equation. The equation in the exponential form is

$$k = Ae^{-Ea/RT} \quad \text{... (37)}$$

where k = specific rate of degradation (i.e. reaction velocity constant)

A = frequency factor (Arrhenius factor)

E_a = energy of activation

R = gas constant

T = absolute temperature

The frequency factor is a measure of frequency of collisions that may be expected between the reacting molecules.

Energy of activation (or heat of activation) refers to the energy required for effective collision to cause a reaction between molecules.

Expressing the equation in logarithmic form

$$\ln k = -\frac{Ea}{RT} + \ln A \quad \text{... (38)}$$

Converting to common logarithmic form:

$$\log k = \frac{-Ea}{2.303\,R} \cdot \frac{1}{T} + \log A \qquad \text{... (40)}$$

where $\log A$ is a constant

If log of k values is plotted against the reciprocal of temperature$(1/T)$, it yields a straight line (Fig. 5.2)

Then the slope is given by $-\frac{\Delta Ea}{2.303\,R}$ and from this value, the heat of reaction can be calculated.

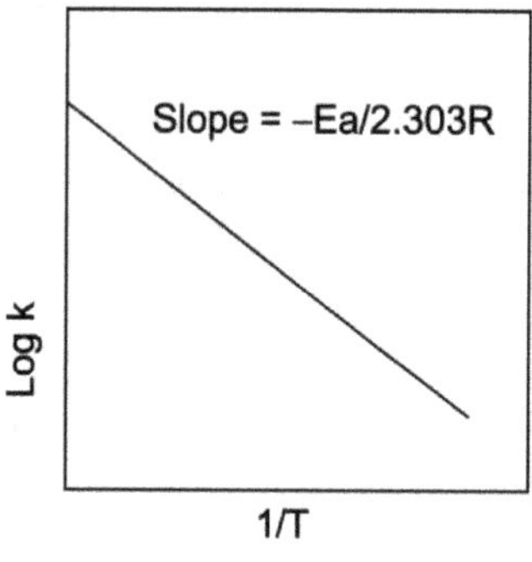

Fig. 5.2

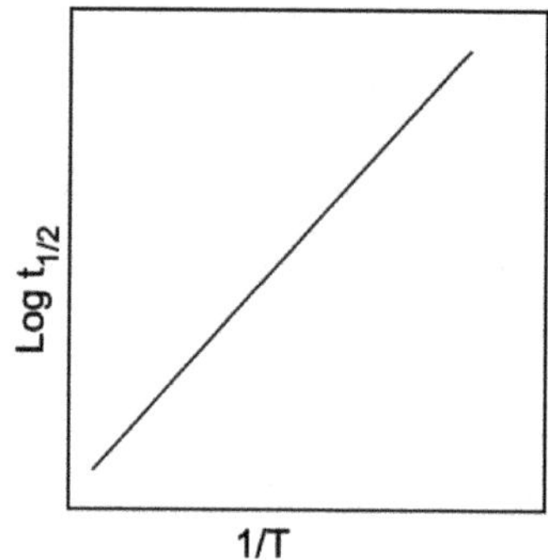

Fig. 5.3

It is also possible to obtain the value of Ea by plotting $\log t_{1/2}$ against $\frac{1}{T}$ (Fig. 5.3)

$$t_{1/2} = \frac{0.693}{k}$$

Or,

$$\log t_{1/2} = \log 0.693 - \log k \qquad \text{... (41)}$$

Thus, on substitution in equation (40) yields

$$\log t_{1/2} = \log 0.693 - \log A + \frac{Ea}{2.303R} \cdot \frac{1}{T}$$

$$\log t_{1/2} = \frac{Ea}{2.303R} \cdot \frac{1}{T} + constant$$

where $(\log 0.693\ and - \log A)$ are constants

A straight line is obtained by plotting $t_{1/2}$ against $1/T$. The slope of the line is equal to $\frac{Ea}{2.303R}$ and from this Ea can be calculated.

Ea may also be obtained by writing equation (40) for two different temperatures and substracting as follows

At a temperature t_2, the equation (40) is given as

$$\log k_2 = \frac{Ea}{2.303R} \cdot \frac{1}{T_2} + \log A \quad \text{... (43)}$$

At a temperature t_1, the equation 40 is given as

$$\log k_1 = -\frac{Ea}{2.303R} \cdot \frac{1}{T_1} + \log A \quad \text{... (44)}$$

where $t_2 > t_1$

On subtraction of equation (43) from (44), we obtain

$$\log \frac{k_2}{k_1} = \frac{E_a}{2.303R} \left(\frac{T_2 - T_1}{T_2 T_1} \right) \quad \text{... (45)}$$

This temperature dependency relationship is useful when the heat of activation (energy of activation) is in the range of 10 to 30 k.cal / mole (*solvolytic process*). If Ea is only 2 to 3 k.cal / mole (*diffusion* or *photolysis*) little advantage is gained. In the same way if the heat of activation is 50 to 70 k.cal / mole (*pyrolysis of polyhydroxylic substances*), the rate of degradation is so fast that it becomes difficult to make use of this relationship.

Arrhenius equation is only an empiric relation and it gives the effect of temperature on an observed rate constant. The temperature dependence especially of uni- and bi-molecular reactions appears to reflect a fundamental physical requirement that must be satisfied for the occurrence of a reaction.

Collision theory: The physical requirement is given by collision state theory or simply collision theory. According to this theory a collision must occur (at a particular temperature) between molecules for a reaction to take place. Further, the collision must be effective i.e., a reaction between molecules does not take place unless the molecules are of certain energy. Thus, the rate of reaction can be considered proportional to the number of molecules of a reactant having sufficient energy. From this it may be understood that all collisions will not lead to reaction and only those collisions with sufficient energy are effective leading to a reaction. If `$Z$' is the collision number (it is the number of collisions per second per cubic centimeter) and $P$, the probability factor (it takes into account that not every collision between molecules does lead to reaction), then, combining the both gives the Arrhenius factor `A' (i.e., $Z + P = A$) and is termed the frequency factor and it refers to the frequency of collisions between molecules. E_a is the minimum kinetic energy a molecule must possess to undergo a reaction.

Transition state theory: It is an alternative to the collision theory. According to this theory, there is equilibrium between the normal reactant molecules and the activated complex of these reacting molecules. Decomposition of this activated complex yields the product. But in this, the amount of energy required for a reaction may be less. For an elementary bimolecular process the reaction may be written as

A + B	[A...B]*	⟶	P
Normal reactant molecules	Activated complex (i.e. activated reactant molecules in transition state)		Product molecule

2. Ionic Strength

Ionic strength of a solution may influence the rate of degradation in accordance with the equation.

$$\log k = \log k_0 + 1.02\, Z_A\, Z_B \sqrt{\mu} \quad \text{... (46)}$$

Z_A and Z_B = charges carried by the reactants A and B in solution respectively

k =the rate constant of degradation

k_0 = the rate constant at infinite dilution.

μ is the ionic strength which is defined as half the sum of the terms obtained by multiplying the molar concentration of each of the ionic species Z_A and Z_B present in solution by square of its valence and may be given as

$$\mu = \frac{1}{2}\,\Sigma\, C_A\, Z_A^2 \text{ and } \mu = \frac{1}{2}\,\Sigma C_B \,.\, Z_B^2 \quad \text{... (47)}$$

If $\log k$ is plotted against μ, the following curves may be obtained. (Fig.5.4) Three possibilities are there for an increase in the ionic strength. When the reactant is positively charged (1) and is undergoing hydrogen ion catalysis, an increase in ionic strength (by the addition of electrolytes such as sodium chloride) produces an increase in the rate of reaction (i.e., k is increased). If one of the reactants is a neutral molecule (2) an increase in ionic strength does not affect the rate of reaction and hence it is independent of ionic strength. The third possibility is that an increase in ionic strength decreases the rate of reaction when positively charged reactant undergoes hydroxyl ion catalysis (3).

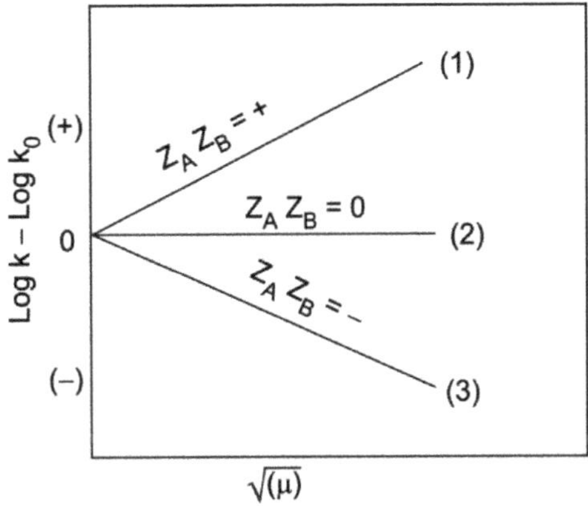

Fig. 5.4

3. Solvent Effect

Hydrolysis is due to reaction with water. Therefore replacement of water with non-aqueous solvents such as alcohol, propylene glycol has often been used. This replacement of a part or all of the water is undertaken to reduce decomposition by hydrolysis. For example, elixir of phenobarbitone contains glycerin and alcohol. Hydrolysis of aspirin is reduced in alcohol-propylene glycol. However, there may be hydrolysis even in the presence of non-aqueous solvents such as alcohol. For example, cyclamic acid degrades at a faster rate in non-aqueous vehicle than in aqueous vehicle.

It may be said that degradation depends on the relative solubilities of the reactants and the degradation products in a given solvent system, dielectric constant of the solvent system and the chemical nature of the reactant species.

The quantitative relationship between the reaction velocity constant of degradation and the solubility is given by the equation considering a reaction.

$$A + B \longrightarrow \underset{\text{(activated complex)}}{(A...B)^*} \longrightarrow \text{products}$$

$$\log k = \log k_0 + \frac{V}{2.303R} \cdot \frac{1}{T} (\Delta\delta_A + \Delta\delta_B - \Delta\delta^*) \quad \text{... (48)}$$

Where k = *observed reaction velocity constant*

k_0 = *reaction velocity constant in an infinitely dilute solution exhibiting ideal behaviour.*

V = *an approximation for the molar volumes of the reactants A and B and the activated complex formed during the reaction and prior to the formation of the products.*

δ_A, δ_B *and* δ^* = *the solubility parameters or internal pressures of the reactants* A, B *and the activated complex respectively*

It is assumed that the properties of the activated complex and the products are similar and therefore $\Delta\delta^*$ *may be taken as the difference in polar characteristics between the solvent and the products. The* $\delta^* = 0$ *indicates similar polar characteristics between the solvent and the products and the* δ_A *and* $\delta_B = 0$ *indicates similar polar characteristics between the solvent and the reactants. If* $\Delta\delta^* = 0$ *and* $\Delta\delta_A + \Delta\delta_B > 0$, *(i.e. polar characteristics are dissimilar), the term* $\frac{V}{2.303RT} (\delta_A + \delta_B - \delta^*)$ *will be positive. Then the reaction velocity* (k) *will be greater than that in an ideal solution. On the other hand, if* $\delta_A + \delta_B = 0$, *and* $\delta^* > 0$, *then the term* $\frac{V}{2.303RT} (\delta_A + \delta_B - \delta^*)$ *will have a negative value indicating lower reaction velocity* (k) *than in the case of an ideal solution.*

In general, it may be said that the solvents which are highly polar will accelerate the reactions that yield products with greater polar characteristics than the reactants (i.e. yield products with higher solubility than that of the reactants). If the products formed have less polar characteristics than that of the reactants (i.e. if the reactants are more soluble than the products) then, the reaction rate will be retarded by solvents of high polarity and accelerated by solvents of low polarities.

4. Dielectric Constant

It has been already mentioned that the dielectric constant has an influence on the reaction rates. Dielectric constant is a property of liquid solvents and therefore the dielectric constant of the solvents affect the rate of hydrolytic reaction and the effect depends on the presence or the absence of an electric charge on the reactant molecule.

If the hydrolytic degradation involves a charged reactant molecule as well another ionic species (H^+ or OH^-) in the system, then the quantitative expression explaining the effect of dielectric constant on reaction rate may be given as

$$ln\, k = ln\, k_{\varepsilon = \infty} - \frac{NZ_AZ_Be^2}{RTr^*}\frac{1}{\varepsilon} \quad \text{... (49)}$$

Where k = *observed reaction rate in a solvent of dielectric constant* **

$k_{\varepsilon = \infty}$ = *reaction rate constant in a solvent of infinite dielectric constant.*

N = *Avagodro's number.*

Z_A *and* Z_B = *charges on the two ionic species (the charged reactant and H^+ or OH^- species).*

e = *value of charge (i.e., the unit of electric charge)*

r^* = *distance between the ionic species in the activated complex.*

If $\ln k$ *is plotted against* $\frac{1}{\epsilon}$, *it yields a straight line. If* Z_A *and* Z_B *carry similar charges, the slope of the line will be negative and hence a decrease in dielectric constant of the solvent will result in a decrease in the rate of hydrolytic degradation. A decrease in dielectric constant can be caused by the addition of a non-aqueous solvent such as ethyl alcohol or propylene glycol or by the replacement of aqueous solvent with non-aqueous solvent in part or in whole.*

If Z_A *and* Z_B *carry opposite charges, the straight line obtained by plotting* $\ln k$ *against* $\frac{1}{\epsilon}$ *will be positive. In this instance, a decrease in dielectric constant will result in an increase in the hydrolytic degradation.*

If the reactant (drug) is a dipole carrying no charge (i.e., neutral molecule) and is involved in a reaction with an ion, the relationship between dielectric constant and the reaction velocity constant is given by

$$ln\, k = ln\, k_{\epsilon = \infty} + \frac{NZ_A^2\, e^2}{2RT}\left(\frac{1}{r_a} - \frac{1}{r^*}\right)\frac{1}{\epsilon} \qquad ...(50)$$

Where, Z_A *= the charge on the ionic hydrolytic species*

r_a *= the radius of the ionic species*

r^* *= the radius of the activated complex.*

As before, if $\ln k$ *is plotted against* $\frac{1}{\epsilon}$*, a straight line is produced.* r^* *being the radius of activated complex (i.e., combined radius of the dipole and the ion) is always larger than* r_a *and hence the slope of the line will always be positive. Therefore* $\ln k$ *will increase on increasing* $\frac{1}{\epsilon}$*. That means between the ion and neutral molecule a decrease in the dielectric constant of the solvent system will only increase the rate of reaction between the ion and the neutral molecule.*

For example, degradation of the antibiotic, chloramphenicol catalyzed by hydrogen ion (H^+) in water-propylene glycol was found to increase on decreasing the dielectric constant of the solvent system by increasing the concentration of propylene glycol. However, the replacement of water by other solvents is frequently employed in pharmacy to stabilize drugs against possible hydrolysis though there is a small increase in degradation rate which may be outweighed by enhancement of solubility of the drug in the solvent of lower dielectric constant.

5. Specific Acid-base catalysis

Hydrolytic degradation is catalyzed by hydrogen (H^+) or hydroxyl (OH^-) ions. The magnitude of the rate of degradation is dependent on pH. Hydrogen ion catalysis dominates at lower pH ranges (i.e., at higher concentrations of hydrogen ion) whereas hydroxyl ion catalysis predominates at higher pH range (i.e. at higher concentration of hydroxyl ions). The degradation rate can be independent of pH at intermediate pH range. Thus, the degradation reaction is said to occur by acid-base catalysis when the rate law for such an accelerated degradation is found to contain a term that involves the concentration of hydrogen ions $[H^+]$ or the concentration of hydroxyl ions $[OH^-]$.

The rate of degradation product formation, $\frac{dp}{dt}$ *dependent on specific acid-base catalysis, may be given for an ester in terms of the general rate law as below.*

$$\frac{dp}{dt} = (k_0 + k_1 [H^+] + k_2 [OH^-][S] \qquad \dots (51)$$

where k_0 *= rate constant for solvent catalytic effect*

k_1 *= rate constant for specific hydrogen ion effect*

k_2 *= rate constant for specific hydroxyl ion effect*

$[S]$ *= solvent concontration.*

For this, the observed reaction rate constant (k_{obs}) *is given by*

$$k_{obs} = k_0 + k_1 [H^+] + k_2 [OH^-] \qquad \dots (52)$$

At low pH, the hydrogen ion concentration is high and hence $k_1 [H^+]$ *is greater than* k_0 *or* $k_2 [OH^-]$*. Then the observed reaction rate constant is given by*

$$k_{obs} = k_1 [H^+] \qquad \dots (53)$$

and in this case specific hydrogen ion catalysis is observed.

At high pH, the hydroxyl ion concentration is high and hence $k_2 [OH^-]$ *is greater than* k_0 *or* k_1*. The equation is then written as*

$$k_{obs} = k_2 [OH^-] \qquad \dots (54)$$

and in this case, specific hydroxyl ion catalysis is observed.

At intermediate pH, or if the products of $k_1 [H^+]$ *and* $k_2 [OH^-]$ *are small in value, the equation is written as*

$$k_{obs} = k_0 \qquad \dots (55)$$

and in this case, the reaction is solvent catalysed.

If the reaction medium is slightly acidic, both the solvent and the specific hydrogen ion (acid) catalysis are involved. On the other hand, if the reaction medium is slightly alkaline, both the solvent and the specific hydroxyl ion (base) catalysis are involved in the degradation process.

The influence of pH on degradation can be determined by measuring the degradation at several hydrogen ion concentrations and obtaining a plot of log of rate constant ($\log k$) versus pH. The point of inflection of such a plot represents the pH of optimum stability.

6. General Acid-base catalysis

Buffers are commonly employed in the formulation of pharmaceutical liquids to maintain the pH of the solution. Though the pH is maintained constant at an optimum level, one or more of the components of the buffer can catalyze the degradation and the reaction is said to be subject to general acid-base catalysis. If the catalytic component is acidic, it is general acid catalysis and if the catalytic component is basic, it is general base catalysis. Common buffer salts which have been found to have catalytic effects are acetates, phosphates and borates.

In order to determine whether a particular pharmaceutical liquid product is catalysed by the buffer system employed, the ionic strength and the ratio of the buffer components (to keep the pH constant) are kept constant while the concentration of the buffer component is altered. If degradation occurs at different concentrations (instead of maintenance of the pH constant) of the buffer components, the reaction is said to be subject to general acid base catalysis. In that case, keeping the ratio of buffer components constant, the concentration of buffer components should be kept as low as possible to minimize the catalytic effect of the buffer components. General acid-base catalysis is to be anticipated, if there is evidence of a significant solvent catalysis.

7. Catalysis

Often chemical reactions are catalyzed by catalysts as already mentioned. A catalyst is a substance which alters the speed of a reaction without itself being altered chemically. A catalyst does not alter the equilibrium of a reversible reaction but speeds up the reaction to attain equilibrium at a shorter time. A catalyst remains unaltered chemically at the end of a reaction.

A catalyst is considered to combine with the reactant and form an activated intermediate complex which then decomposes to regenerate the catalyst and yields the product. Catalysis is also considered to occur at the surface of the catalyst in the case of heterogeneous catalysis.

8. Light

Light induces chemical reactions. Radiations of proper frequency must be absorbed to cause a chemical reaction (degradation). Photochemical decompositions do not depend on temperature for activation of molecules. These reactions are usually complex and proceed by a series of steps.

Stabilization of medicinal agents

Pharmaceutical preparations or products often may exhibit physical or chemical reactions and that may end in instability. Due to such instability, the preparation gets deteriorated. This deterioration may lead to

(a) reduction in the activity of a preparation

(b) formation of toxic products

(c) an inelegant product.

Apart from these effects, microbial contamination also may cause deterioration of the product. Ultimately the product becomes unacceptable.

Hence it is necessary to perform stability testing to find out the extent of deterioration or degradation and to ensure the degradation has not exceeded an acceptable level assuring,

1. the safety of the patient and
2. the therapeutic activity of the product

Decomposition or degradation of active ingredients (drug substances) in pharmaceutical preparations may occur by hydrolysis, oxidation-reduction, racemization, decarboxylation, ring cleavage, photolysis, isomerization and epimerization.

Physical degradation of pharmaceutical products may be due to loss of water, loss of volatile constituents, absorption of water, crystal growth, polymorphic changes, and colour changes.

However, the degradative reactions leading to chemical instability in pharmaceutical products are mainly the hydrolysis and oxidation-reduction.

1. Hydrolysis

Many pharmaceutical preparations contain esters or amide functional groups that undergo hydrolysis in solution. Hydrolysis is a reaction of an ester or amide with water. Though hydrolysis can occur with pure water, the presence of a catalyst which supplies hydrogen (H^+) ions or hydroxyl ions (OH^-), is needed to promote the reaction.

The ester hydrolysis whether acid catalyzed or alkali catalyzed can in general, be represented as follows:

$$\underset{\text{ester}}{R'-\overset{\overset{\displaystyle O}{\|}}{C}-OR} + H_2O \qquad \underset{\text{acid}}{R'-\overset{\overset{\displaystyle O}{\|}}{C}-OH} + \underset{\text{alcohol}}{HOR}$$

This reaction denotes second order reaction. However, it is possible to treat this as *pseudo* - first order reaction by keeping H^+ or OH^- at a considerably higher concentration or by keeping H^+ or OH^- concentrations essentially constant by the use of buffers.

In the study of degradation of drugs by ester hydrolysis, first order kinetic expressions have been employed whenever possible.

The drugs which undergo ester hydrolysis may be procaine, atropine, aspirin etc.

Amide hydrolysis is similar to ester hydrolysis but it forms an amine instead of an alcohol. It may be represented as follows:

$$\underset{\text{amide}}{R-\overset{\overset{\displaystyle O}{\|}}{C}-\overset{\overset{\displaystyle H}{|}}{N}-R'} + H_2O \qquad R-\overset{\overset{\displaystyle O}{\|}}{C}-OH + \underset{\text{amine}}{H_2\cdot N-R'}$$

Examples of amides that undergo amide hydrolysis are niacinamide, phenethicillin, chloramphenicol, barbiturates, penicillins etc.

Amides have, in general, greater stability than the structurally similar esters.

Ring alteration: Hydrolytic reactions may also proceed by ring cleavage with subsequent attack by H^+ or OH^- ions. Examples of drugs which undergo hydrolysis by ring alteration are hydrochlorothiazide, pilocarpine and reserpine.

Protection against Hydrolysis

Pharmaceutical liquid preparations containing water are the most susceptible to hydrolysis, e.g., solutions, suspensions and emulsions. Solid dosage forms such as tablets and granules may also undergo hydrolysis because of entry of water vapor from the atmosphere or because of water of crystallization in other ingredients.

Hydrolysis of drug products such as powders, granules, tablets and capsules may be prevented by avoiding contact with water vapor. It involves the control of atmospheric humidity during preparation, purification, and packaging. Extra protection can be achieved by way of including porous envelopes containing desiccants (like silica gels) in the containers.

In the case of liquid dosage forms, the method of protection is by reducing the rate of hydrolysis. This may be achieved by adjusting the pH to an optimum level at which the catalytic effects of H^+ or OH^- ions (specific acid base catalysis) are at a minimum by the inclusion of proper buffer solutions.

If the hydrolytic degradation is general acid-base catalyzed i.e. by the acid and basic species (i.e. acid and its conjugate base) of the buffer solution in addition to H^+ or OH^-, the buffer concentration should be kept at a minimum.

Hydrolytic reactions may in general be minimized by partial or full replacement of water (i.e. by a reduction in dielectric constant) with a solvent of lower dielectric constants such as alcohol, glycol, glucose and mannitol solutions.

Complexation is also a method by which hydrolytic reactions may be inhibited. For example, benzocaine is protected against hydrolysis by forming a molecular complex of benzocaine with caffeine.

By modification of chemical structure by increasing the length of or by branching the acyl or alkyl groups, the rate of hydrolysis of an ester may be decreased owing to stearic hinderance.

Hydrolysis is a solvolysis reaction and hence the degradation by hydrolysis depends on solubility of the drug. Hence, by reducing the solubility of the drug by forming less soluble salt or ester of the drug, hydrolysis can be decreased. For example, insoluble chlorthiazide (may be formulated as suspension) is less prone to hydrolysis than its soluble sodium salt. Solvolysis can be reduced by preparing difficultly soluble esters and other derivatives. For example, chloramphenicol palmitate is difficultly soluble ester which can be formulated as suspension.

Erythromycin is an antibiotic. It gets degraded in the acidic environment as found in stomach. To protect the drug, erythromycin is converted into an ester. The ester remains inactive until the drug is released from the ester by enzymatic hydrolysis in the body (prodrug concept).

Sterile dry powders (penicillin powder) or dry syrups (ampicillin syrup) are prepared and dispensed to exclude water till it is used and at the time of usage, they are reconstituted with water for injection or purified water respectively. This is to avoid hydrolytic decomposition.

2. Oxidation - reduction

The instability of a considerable number of pharmaceutical preparations are due to oxidative decomposition of active ingredients. Oxidation involves the addition of oxygen or the removal of hydrogen. Oxidation and reduction occur simultaneously. A substance is said to be oxidized if one or more electrons are removed from it. The simplest type of oxidation involves the removal of an electron. For example, ferrous ion is oxidized to ferric ion by the elimination of an electron.

$$Fe^{++} \longrightarrow Fe^{+++} + 1e$$

Autoxidation is the most common form of oxidative decomposition that occurs in many of the pharmaceutical preparations and it involves a free radial chain process. The rancidity occurring in fixed oils is due to autoxidation during storage.

Autoxidation is a reaction of a substance with molecular oxygen (present in air) and it involves free radical chain process. The autoxidation of an organic substance may be simply represented as follows:

Chain initiation: It is induced by benzoyl peroxide or ultra violet light or heat in which free radicals are produced.

$$RH \xrightarrow{hv} \underset{\text{free radical}}{R^0 + (H)}$$

Chain propagation:

$$R^o + O_2 \longrightarrow RO_2^o$$

$$RO_2^o + RH \longrightarrow RO^o + OH^o + R^o$$

Chain termination:

$$R^0 + HI \longrightarrow \underset{\text{(stable free radical)}}{RH + I^0}$$

$$RO_2^0 + X \longrightarrow \underset{\text{(termination by inhibitor)}}{\text{inactive products}}$$

where *HI* and *X* are chain inhibitors.

$$\left.\begin{array}{l} R^0 + R^0 \\ RO_2^0 + RO_2^0 \\ RO_2^0 + R^0 \end{array}\right\} \longrightarrow \begin{array}{c} \text{inactive products} \\ \text{(self termination)} \end{array} \begin{array}{l} R-R \\ RO_2-RO_2 \\ RO_2-R \end{array}$$

In an autoxidative degradation, only a small amount of oxygen is needed to initiate the reaction and thereafter oxygen concentration is relatively unimportant.

Heavy metals such as copper, ion, cobalt, and nickel catalyze the oxidative degradation (For e.g. oxidation of ascorbic acid is catalyzed by copper ions).

Many oxidative degradations are catalyzed by hydrogen and hydroxyl ions.

Some solvents other than water may have a catalyzing effect on oxidations. For example, aldehydes, ethers, and ketones may cause free radical reactions.

The kinetics of overall oxidative degradation processes are influenced by heat and light. The degradation of pharmaceutical substances by oxidative degradation follows first order or second order kinetic expressions.

Some drugs that undergo oxidative decomposition are ergometrine, epinephrine, heparin, paraldehyde, tetracyclines, vitamin D, K, C etc.

Protection against oxidation

Most oxidative degradation of pharmaceutical compounds are probably autoxidative and hence antioxidants that are effective against atmospheric oxygen are often used to provide protection against autoxidation. They may be ultraviolet absorbers such as phenyl salicylate and 2-hydroxy benzophenone; hydroperoxide destroyers such as organic compounds of sulphur and phosphorous; metal deactivators (by complexation) such as chelating agents like citric acid, ethylene diamine tetra acetic acid (EDTA) and 8 hydroxy quinone; and chain terminating agents (antioxidants) such as butyl hydroxy anisole (BHA), nor-dihydro guariaretic acid (NDGA) and gallic acid esters such as propyl and $n-$ butyl gallates.

The effectiveness of antioxidants can be increased through the use of synergists such as chelating agents and it also depends on the concentrations used, the solution pH and packaging.

When oxidation is catalyzed by hydrogen and hydroxyl ion, the pH of optimum stability must be ensured.

Water soluble antioxidants act by undergoing oxidation in preference to the drug. Oil soluble antioxidants prevent free radical chain processes.

Antioxidants commonly used for aqueous systems are sodium bisulfite, sodium sulfite, sodium metabisulfate, ascorbic acid, thioglycerol etc.

Antioxidants commonly used for oil systems are ascorbyl palmitate, hydroquinone, propyl gallate butylated hydroxy anisole (BHA), $\alpha-$ tocopherol and butylated hydroxy toulene (BHT).

Oxidation of fats and oils may be retarded by hydrogenation. Drugs which are attacked by atmospheric oxygen may be protected by replacing the air in the container with an inert gas. For example, ergometrine injection is protected against oxidation by replacing the air with inert gas nitrogen in the ampoules.

An effective antioxidation (preservation against oxidation) can be obtained by taking into account some three or four factors. For example, drug substances such as ascorbic acid and epinephrine (adrenaline) may be stabilized by excluding oxygen, buffering the solutions to a favorable pH, using metal-free solvents, adding chain inhibitors, excluding light and storing at a low temperature.

3. Photolytic decomposition

Chemical reactions produced directly or indirectly by means of light are called photochemical reactions. In this, the molecules are activated by photons (the energy unit of radiation is known as photon and is equivalent to one *quantum* of energy) of high energy radiations like visible rays, ultraviolet rays, X-rays, γ – rays or any other part of electromagnetic spectrum. Reaction between hydrogen and chlorine is a classic example of photochemical reaction. The energy of a photon $\boldsymbol{E}$ is given by

$$\boldsymbol{E = hv = \frac{hc}{\lambda}}$$

Where, $\boldsymbol{h}$ = Plank's constant (6.62×10^{-27})

$\boldsymbol{v}$ = Frequency of radiant energy

$\boldsymbol{c}$ = velocity of radiation in vacuum, 3×10^{10}cmsec^{-1}

One Einstein of a visible light of wavelength 6000Ā has energy equal to 45 k. calories/mole. Hence, absorption of radiations in the visible or ultraviolet region can induce a chemical reaction by breaking a chemical bond or high energy reactive complex. The infra-red has practically no effect on chemical reaction. The X-rays and λ- rays are associated with so much energy that they can induce ionization reactions.

A photochemical reaction in which series of reactions are set up and millions of molecules react for each quantum of light absorbed is called chain reaction in which a high quantum yield is obtained. However, presence of traces of foreign materials (inhibitors) can retard the chain reaction. *Example: – combination of hydrogen and chlorine.* Certain reactants which are not sensitive to light are made sensitive in the presence of a small quantity of a foreign substance which absorb light and stimulate the reaction without taking part in the chemical reaction. Example: – *decomposition of ozone into oxygen is photosensitized by chlorine.*

These reactions are usually complex and proceed by a series of steps.

Pharmaceutical compounds which undergo photochemical decomposition are riboflavin, phenothiazines, nifedipine, chlordiazepoxide, furosemide etc.

Exposure to light may produce oxidation-reduction, ring rearrangement or modification and polymerization. The shorter the wave length of light, the greater is the effect of light in initiating the chemical reaction because of higher energy.

A photochemical reaction may be accompanied by a thermal reaction. However, this thermal reaction is entirely different in character from that of ordinary thermal reaction. The thermal reaction once induced by light may continue after the light source has been withdrawn. The energy available in photochemical reaction is much greater than in a normal thermal reaction. The possible orders of photochemical reactions are second order, first order and zero-order. Few drugs which are affected by light are Nifedipine, chlordiazepoxide, and furosemide.

Protection against photolytic degradation: Photochemical reactions can be reduced by storing the product in darkness. Amber-colored bottles are used to minimize these reactions. Packaging the bottled liquid in cartons also act as a physical barrier to light.

DL methionine was found to have photostabilizing effect on ascorbic acid solution buffered by phosphate and not by citrate at pH 4.5. Uric acid was found to produce a photoprotective effect in buffered and unbuffered solution of sulphathiazole sodium.

Some measures may be preserving the drugs in dark places, shady places, hermitically sealed metal containers, in amber-colored glass containers or vials or ampoules, by using ultraviolet stabilizers (as part of the glass containers composition) which absorb ultraviolet radiation and dispose of energy without forming free- radicals. Example- phenyl salicylate and 2-hydroxyl benzophenone. Tablets can be protected against light by strip packing.

British Pharmaceutical Codex defines a light resistant container is one that does not transmit more than 15% of radiation between 290 and 450 nm.

Accelerated Stability Testing

If pharmaceutical preparations or new formulations are stored under normal conditions, their instabilities are detectable only after long storage periods. Such a method is time consuming and uneconomical. In an attempt to reduce the time required to obtain information on instabilities, various tests are undertaken. These tests involve storage of the preparations under conditions that will accelerate decomposition at a faster rate. As there is rapid deterioration when stored under conditions that place a higher stress or challenge to the preparations, the instability becomes detectable at a short period.

The most common stresses often used is the temperature (i.e., elevated temperatures). It is mainly applicable for drugs in solutions, The other stresses may be humidity and light or any other stress related to a particular preparation.

The objectives of accelerated stability testing may be

1. the best formulation from a series of different initial formulations may be selected because rapid detection of decomposition is made possible.
2. it is useful to predict the shelf-life of a product (i.e., to predict the expiry date).
3. it provides for a rapid means of quality control.

Prediction of shelf-life (fixing of expiration date)

Shelf-life is the period during which a pharmaceutical dosage form keeps its qualities. The predication of shelf-life is based on applying the Arrhenius equation which gives the effect of temperature on rate constant, k of a chemical reaction.

Fortunately, it is not required for the purpose of stability prediction to determine the mechanism of degradation. The stability of any active component in a pharmaceutical preparation can be evaluated by determining some property of the degradation (such as colour disappearance, concentration) under accelerated storage conditions as a function of time. If this function can be linearised with any of the chemical kinetic reaction orders (i.e., it refers to the determination of the order of reaction), temperature dependency of the degradation can be obtained with the help of Arrhenius equation. Then it is possible to determine the chemical stability of the active ingredient for an extended shelf-storage period under normal conditions of storage. In other words, the period during which the preparation will remain stable under normal conditions of storage can be determined.

Consider a multi-sulphanomide preparation whose instability is measured in terms of colour disappearance. The preparation is subjected to different elevated temperatures say 40°C, 50°C, 60°C, 70°C and 80°C to accelerate the degradation (measured in terms of colour intensity decrease). Plots of changes in absorbance at 500 nm (measured by the use of photocolorimeter) for each elevated temperatures against time are obtained (Fig. 5.5). Such a plot shows that changes in absorbance versus time is linear as shown in the figure.

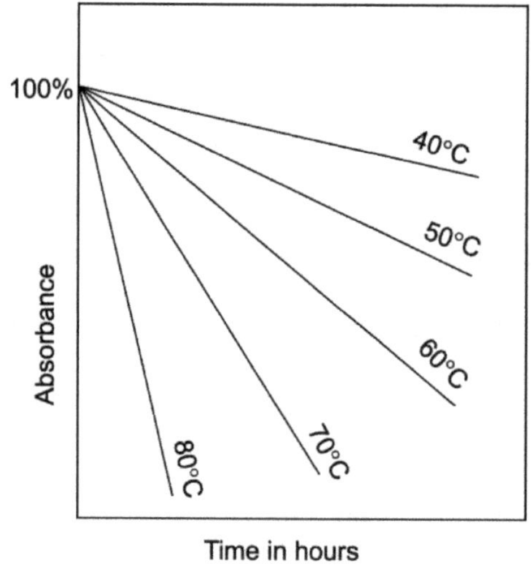

Fig. 5.5

The linear curves obtained for different elevated temperatures show that colour loss is following zero order kinetics in accordance with the equation.

$$A_t = A_0 - kt$$

where A_t = absorbance at time t

A_0 = absorbance at time zero i.e. initial absorbance

k = rate constant.

The slopes of the lines represent the rate of change in colour with time for different temperatures and the value of k, for each temperature can be obtained from the respective slope. The k value becomes greater and greater as the temperature is increased.

Then, an Arrhenius plot of $\log k$ values versus the reciprocal of the absolute temperature (T) is obtained. Such a plot may be shown in Fig. 5.6.

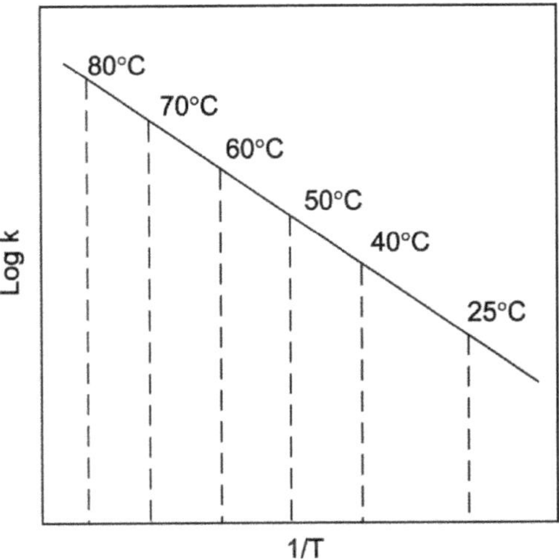

Fig. 5.6

Since the plot is linear, the stability of the preparation may be predicted at ordinary room temperature by extrapolating the curve to the lower temperature say 25°C. The k value is then read out for the lower temperature (say 25°C) and from this value, the shelf life period may be calculated using zero-order kinetic equation, $A_t = A_0 - kt$

For example, in order to predict the time for the absorbance to fall from 0.470 (A_0) at time zero to 0.225 (A_t) at time t, representing the potency of the preparation has fallen below the desired level for use, the zero order reaction is used. Assume at 25°C, the rate constant is 2.09×10^{-5} hr^{-1}.

Using zero order equation,

$$A_t = A_0 - kt$$

$$kt = -A_t + A_0$$

$$t = \frac{-A_t + A_0}{k}$$

and substituting the values, the shelf-life period is given as

$$t = \frac{(-0.225 + 0.470)}{2.09 \times 10^{-5}}$$

= **11722 hours or 488 days or 1 year 4 months.**

The shelf-life period is nearly 1 year 4 months.

Suppose the concentration is measured as a function of time at different elevated temperatures and the degradation (shown by a decrease in concentration) follows first order kinetics, the shelf life period can be calculated as shown in the example that follows.

Suppose the initial concentration is 90 units / ml and the specific decomposition rate k is obtained by using Arrhenius plot is 3.63×10^{-5} hr^{-1} at room temperature 25°C. Suppose the concentration falls below 40 units / ml, it is not potent for use. Then the expiration date can be predicted considering the date of manufacture.

The initial concentration (c) at time zero is 90 units / ml.

The final concentration c at time `t'is 40 units / ml.

k at 25°C = 3.63×10^{-5} per hour.

Using the first order kinetic equation

$$t = \frac{2.303}{k}.\log\frac{co}{c}$$

and substituting the values

$$t = \frac{2.303}{3.63 \times 10^{-5}} \log\frac{90}{40}$$

= **22344 hrs or 2 years 6 months**

The various steps involved in the prediction of shelf-life may be summarized as follows:

1. The preparation for which the stability is to be determined is divided into 5 or 6 portions and each portion is stored at different temperatures say 40°, 50°, 60°, 70° and 80° in order to accelerate the degradation.

2. Samples from each portion are withdrawn at different intervals of time and determined the remaining concentrations.

3. The order of reaction (whether zero, first or second order) is determined by plotting the appropriate function of the concentration (whether $a, \log(a - x)$ or $1/(a - x)$ against time and the linearship relation is determined (This one is graphical method. Other methods such as half life method or substitution method also can be used).

4. From the slopes of the lines, the reaction velocity constant k for the degradation at each of the elevated temperatures is calculated. (See Fig. 5.5)

5. Employing the Arrhenius relationship, the reaction velocity constant k for the degradation at room temperature (generally 25°C) is determined. This may be obtained from the linear plot of the logarithm of the k values for various elevated temperatures against the reciprocals of absolute temperatures and then extrapolating the curve to 25°C and reading off the k value at 25°C (See Fig.5.6)

6. The k value obtained for 25°C is then substituted in the appropriate rate equation (already determined order of reaction) and an estimate is obtained for the time during which the product will remain potent (i.e., shelf-life period).

7. Appropriate calculation is carried out to find out the amount of drug to be added in excess (overage) to compensate for the loss during the shelf-life period to assure 100% concentration in the product during use within its shelf-life period especially for vitamin formulations.

A similar method with some modifications has been suggested. In this method, a plot of log percent of drug remaining versus time in days is obtained as shown in Fig. 5.7.

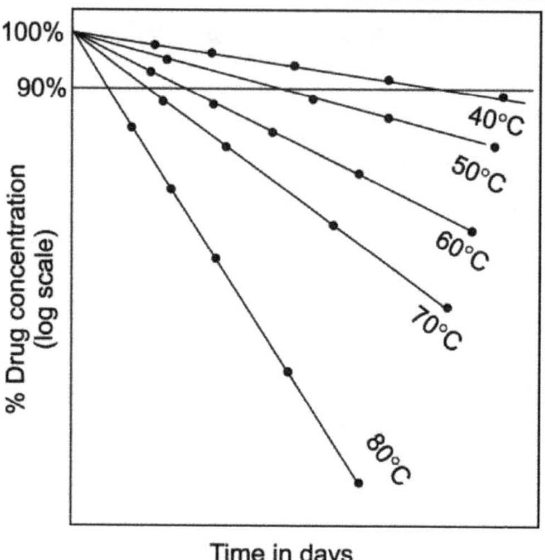

Fig. 5.7

From the above graph, (Fig. 5.7) the time for the potency to fall to 90% of the original value which normally means expiry date is read. Then the log time to 90% versus the reciprocal of either the Celsius or Kelvin scale is plotted as shown in Fig. 5.8.

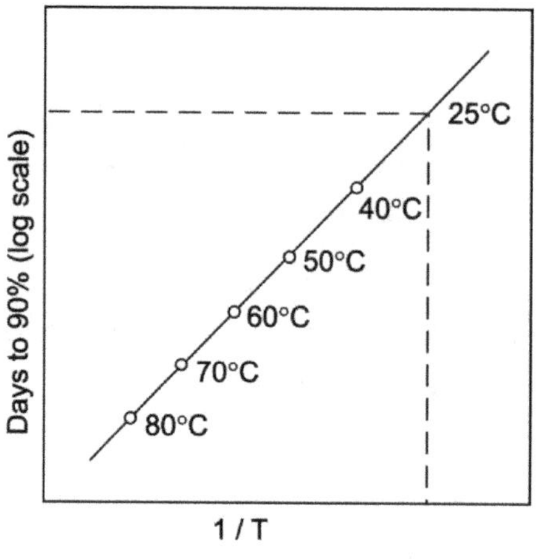

Fig. 5.8

The straight line of the curve is extrapolated to lower temperature (say 25°C) and from this the number of days (which is the shelf-life period) at 25°***C*** is read directly.

An improved technique to evaluate stability by isothermal kinetics has been suggested by Rogers et al. In this technique the energy of activation and reaction velocity constant and the stability prediction are obtained in a single experiment. It involves raising the temperature of a product under test by programming the temperature to change at predetermined rate. Samples are withdrawn and analyzed at suitable time intervals.

Temperature and time are related by

$$\frac{1}{T} = \frac{1}{T_0} + at \qquad \text{... (56)}$$

Or,

$$\frac{1}{T} - \frac{1}{T_0} = at \qquad \text{... (57)}$$

where T_0 is the initial temperature and `$a'$ is the reciprocal heating rate constant and at any time during the run, the Arrhenius equation at time zero and at any time `t' may be given

$$ln\, k_t = ln\, k_0 - \frac{Ea}{R}\left(\frac{1}{T} - \frac{1}{T_0}\right) \qquad \text{... (58)}$$

Substituting for $\frac{1}{T} - \frac{1}{T_0}$, the equation is

$$ln\, k_t = ln\, k_0 - \frac{Ea}{R}\, at \qquad \text{... (59)}$$

Temperature being a function of time t, a measure of stability k_t is directly obtained over a range of temperature.

Overages:

Once the shelf-life has been determined, excess quantity of drug (overage) must be added to the preparation (for e.g., vitamin preparations) to maintain 100% of the labelled amount of the drug during the shelf-life of the product. This can be easily calculated and added to the preparation at the time of manufacture so that 100% of the drug claimed on the label is assured throughout the shelf-life period.

This is not applicable to highly potent drugs. Overages, added in the formulations, should be within the limits compatible with therapeutic requirements and for shelf life period.

Many vitamins degrade at a finite rate when stored under ambient room temperature. To compensate for this finite rate of degradation, it is necessary to add overages during the formulation. Hence manufactures include excess quantities (i.e., overages) at the time of manufacture. The organization of the Pharmaceutical Products of India (OPPI) as well as Federation International Pharmaceutique (FIP) has recommended the overages shown in the following table for various vitamins. The student may find the OPPI overages are in general higher than FIP overages perhaps due to climatic reasons.

Vitamin	**OPPI**			**FIP**		
	Oral liquid in %	**Tablets in %**	**Parenteral products in %**	**Oral liquids in %**	**Oral solids in %**	**Soft capsules in %**
Vitamin A	100	75	50	60	60	75
Vitamin B1	175	100	100	80	50	175
Vitamin B2	150	100	100	80	80	100
Folic acid	100	-	100	50	80	-
Pantothenic acid	100	75	100	80	50	75
Vitamin C	175	-	-	50	-	100
Vitamin D	75	100	80	80	80	60

Limitations of Accelerated Stability Testing

Stability predictions based on Arrhenius equation are valid only when the decomposition is a thermal phenomenon with activation energy of about 10 to 30 k cal / mole.

The prediction may be invalid because at higher temperatures solvent produces unequal moisture concentration. There may be less humidity and oxygen solubility at higher temperatures whereas at room temperatures, there may be more moisture and oxygen content.

There is also a possibility of change in the order of reaction during the period of study. For example a zero order reaction may subsequently become a first order, second order and the activation energy may also change if the decomposition process is a complex process. Thus, there is a possibility that the application of higher stresses may cause reactions that would not take place at lower stresses (actual storage conditions).

During normal storage conditions, formulations are exposed to a variety of weather conditions and temperatures except a few which are stored at a particular temperature in a refrigerator or in a cold room. But in our experiments, the natural weather conditions are not simulated. The test would be more meaningful if it is performed in normal storage conditions.

When temperature is elevated in disperse systems (such as emulsions and suspensions), viscosity is decreased as a result of alterations in physical characteristics and this may introduce large errors in the prediction of stability.

Advantages of Accelerated stability testing

Even with all these difficulties, the accelerated stability testing is acceptable since the predicted shelf lives are sufficiently accurate when the data are analyzed statistically as compared to shelf lives of the product stored under normal conditions.

Determination of the causes of decomposition

The causes of decomposition may be dependent upon

(a) chemical structures of drug substances

(b) chemical structures of decomposition products

(c) the properties of additives used, impurities present if any and the material of the container and

(d) storage conditions

The decomposition may be indicated by the appearance and odour of the preparation. Knowledge of the behavior of similar compounds may also indicate the possible route of decomposition.

However a series of tests may be conducted to rule out the causes or to find out the causes of decompositions. A simple demonstration may help to understand clearly.

Consider a drug solution in water sealed in ampoules divided into six groups, three of which contain inert nitrogen gas in the space above the solution within the ampoules and the remaining consist of oxygen (or air) in the space above the solution within the ampoules. Now the ampoules are exposed to different conditions as shown below:

	Ampoules containing O_2 above the solution	**Ampoule mark**
1.	Exposed to light	A_1
2.	Exposed to heat	A_2
3.	Stored in dark	A_3

	Ampoules containing nitrogen gas above the solution	Ampoule mark
1.	Exposed to light	B_1
2.	Exposed to heat	B_2
3.	Stored in dark	B_3

The contents of ampoules are analyzed, drawn at different time intervals.

The results may be summarized as follows:

(a) Decomposition in all the ampoules irrespective of the ampoules having oxygen or nitrogen above the solution indicates hydrolytic decomposition.

(b) Degradation by oxidation is indicated by the decomposition in only three groups of ampoules (A_1, A_2 and A_3) containing oxygen irrespective of exposure to light, heat or darkness.

(c) A photochemical reaction is indicated by the decomposition only in ampoules A_1 and B_1 groups exposed to light.

(d) Thermal decomposition is indicated by the decomposition only in A_2 and and not in all the other ampoules.

In a similar way, the effect of pH on decomposition of drug solutions can be carried out.

Accelerated Tests for Photochemical stability

Accelerated tests for photochemical stability can be done by inducing rapid decomposition by means of artificial light source of varying intensities simulating the effects of sunlight or room illumination. The relationship between the intensities of light and rate of photo-degradation is a unique function of the formulation under test. In this method, photochemical decomposition is measured quantitatively. Extrapolation of the results to predict the effects of normal storage conditions is often difficult and thus warrants a development of a rational approach. However to overcome the problem of photo-degradation, it is necessary to pack the formulation in amber colored containers (bottles) and to store away from light. An extra protection from light is provided by placing the container in a carton box.

Accelerated tests for physical stability

Physical instabilities are many and are due to varied causes. Hence it is not possible to design a single universal test. However, a general rule can be followed if the formulations are stable under higher stresses, it will be stable under normal conditions.

(a) Accelerated tests for moisture absorption In this method, products are placed in an environment of high relative humidity and controlled temperatures. It is achieved by using a number of small cabinets each containing a different saturated salt solution that produces the desired humidity conditions. Now-a-days sophisticated environmental chambers are available to create required humidities and temperatures. The formulation (tablets, capsules etc) is kept both in packed forms and unpacked forms in the chambers and its physical and chemical stabilities are assessed. The results will indicate whether the product is susceptible to moisture and also whether the container needs to provide a high degree of protection.

(b) Accelerated tests for emulsion stability: An emulsion is prepared in large quantities Small quantities are filled in a number of containers with closures and stored in a range of temperatures from 45° to 70°C. Agitation and decreases in viscosity of the continuous phase lead to increased collisions of dispersed phase. If the emulsion withstands this higher stress, it may be assumed that the emulsion will be stable under normal conditions of storage. The method is not applicable to emulsions containing drugs and emulsifying agents which undergo decomposition at higher temperatures since the conclusion will be erroneous. An alternate and best method is by centrifugation which accelerates rate of creaming in emulsions. The rate of creaming is directly proportional to the speed of ultracentrifuges up to 60,000 rpm. It is possible to predict sufficiently accurately about the creaming problems of majority of emulsions at normal storage conditions.

(c) Accelerated tests for suspension stability: The stability problems with the suspension are settling of solid phase (dispersed phase) and formation of a solid cake. Both are undesirable. Both the problems may be accelerated by centrifugation. High speed centrifugation is not preferable since it produces a close-packed sediment. Low speed centrifugation equivalent to four times the gravitational force is preferred to study the physical stability.

Another stability problem with the suspension is crystal growth. For this study, temperature fluctuations under normal storage conditions are to be simulated. It is done by exposing suspensions between 23° and 33°C using a cycling time of 16 minutes. The cycling is normally repeated hundred times and crystal growth is observed. The crystal growth depends upon the particle concentration, the bulk particle solubility, temperature fluctuation range and the frequency of fluctuation.

Drug decomposition in solid state

The breakdown of drugs in the solid state also occurs which is very important to decide the expiry date of solid dosage forms. Single component solid dosage forms degrade either by zero order or by first order reaction. The decomposition of multi drugs in solid dosage forms is more complex than single component and the decomposition may be zero or first order and sometimes it is difficult to differentiate between the two.

In tablets and other solid dosage forms, there is a possibility of solid-solid interaction which may be between drugs or between drugs and additives. This may be found out by running thin layer chromatography with the drug alone and drug-additive mixture. Any change in the R_f value of the drug indicates drug interaction. The interaction may also be studied by using diffuse reflectance spectroscopy.

Factors like temperature, hydrolysis, oxidation etc., affecting liquid dosage forms also affect solid dosage forms. To protect from these factors, the dosage forms are packed suitably e.g. packing with metal foils, strip packing, putting in amber coloured bottles. Fading of color in tablets on exposure to light (photolysis reaction) in solid dosage forms is another problem. This photolysis was found to be a surface phenomenon. Other problems associated with the solid dosage forms are polymorphic transitions, sublimation and dehydration.

Various experimental methods used in solid state kinetics are reflectance spectroscopy, X-ray diffraction, thermal analysis, microscopy, dilatometry and gas pressure-volume analysis.

ADDENDUM

1. Colloidal dispersion

1. The velocity of migration of an aqueous ferric hydroxide sol toward negative electrode of the electrophoresis cell was found to be 16.5 × 10⁻⁴ cm/sec at 20 °C. The distance between the electrodes in the cell was 20 cm and the applied emf was 110 volts. What is a) the zeta potential of the sol and b) the sign of the charge on the particle?

The electrophoretic mobility $\frac{v}{E}$

$$= \frac{Velocity\ of\ mobility}{Applied\ emf/resistance}$$

$$= \frac{16.5 \times 10^{-4}\ cm/sec}{110\ volts\ /20\ volts\ cm}$$

$$= 3 \times 10^{-4}\ cm^2\ volt^{-1}\ sec^{-1}$$

The zero potential is given by

$$s = 141 \times \frac{V}{E}$$

$$= 141 \times 3 \times 10^{-4}$$

$$= 0.042 \text{ volts or } 42 \text{ milli volts}$$

(For a colloidal system in which water is the medium the coefficient is 141 at 20°C. The coefficient becomes 128 at 25°C.

As the migration of sol is towards negative electrode of the electrophoretic cell. The colloid is positively charged.

2. ***The electrophoretic mobility for bentonite in water is around -3.40×10^{-4} cm/sec per volt cm at 25 °C. The electrophoretic mobility of bismuth subnitrate particles in water at 25 °C is around $+ 2.20 \times 10^{-4}$ cm/sec per volt/cm. calculate the zeta potential of bentonite and of bismuth subnitrate at 25 °C.***

The zeta potential of bentonite particle $= -3.40 \times 10^{-4} \times 128$

(The coefficient of a colloid at 25°C in which water in the medium is 128)

$= -\ 43.5$ milli volts

The potential of bismuth sub nitrate is $2.20 \times 10^{-4} \times 128$

$= 28.2$ milli volts

Donnan effect

The Donnan effect is an important factor in various body fluids. The interstitial fluid of the body lies between the vascular system (i.e., blood plasma and erythrocytes within the blood) and the tissue cells of the body. The plasma and erythrocytes (i.e., blood) contain non-diffusible protein anions, whereas the interstitial fluid contains only diffusible ions such as K^+, Na^+, and Cl^-. Therefore, the Donnan membrane effect in the body is to influence the distribution of the diffusible ions. The protein anions (within the blood vessels) tend to attract and retain small cations (Na^+ and K^+) in the tissue cells and blood vessels, and repel small anions (Cl^-) into the surrounding interstitial fluid.

Body cells ↔ interstitial cells ↔ blood plasma + erythrocytes (blood vessels)

Donnan membrane equilibrium gives the ratio of concentration of diffusible anion (negatively charged ion i.e., the drug ion) outside and inside the membrane at equilibrium. The equation, given below, shows that negatively charged (non-diffusible) polyelectrolyte ions (R^-) inside a semi-permeable sac would influence the concentration of diffusible anion inside and outside the sac. The polyelectrolyte would tend to drive the diffusible drug ion (D^-), carrying the same charge as the electrolyte, out through the membrane. This effect promotes the absorption of drug molecules. For example, if sodium chloride solution (representing the drug solution) is placed on one side of a semi-permeable membrane, and a negatively charged colloid such as sodium carboxy methyl cellulose (a poly electrolyte) solution is placed on other side, the diffusible ions of sodium chloride (Na^+ and Cl^-) and of sodium of the sodium carboxy methyl cellulose (Na^+) can diffuse freely through the semi-permeable membrane but not the colloid particle R^-, i.e., carboxy methyl cellulose. However, at equilibrium, the concentration of positively charged ions in the solution on either side of the membrane must balance the concentration of negatively charged ions and for that the chloride ion (Cl^-) carrying the same charge as that of carboxy methyl cellulose chloride will be pushed to the other side. The equation relating Donnan equilibrium is

$$\frac{[D^-]_o}{[D^-]_i} = \sqrt{1 + \frac{[R^-]_i}{[D^-]_i}} \quad \text{or} \quad \frac{[Cl^-]_o}{[Cl^-]_i} = \sqrt{1 + \frac{[R^-]_i}{[Cl^-]_i}}$$

3. ***Consider a non-diffusible carboxy methyl cellulose (negatively charged ion, say $[R^-]$) is equilibrated across a semi-permeable membrane with a solution of drug, sodium salicylate in which both Na^+ and salicylate ion (negatively charged say $[D^-]$) are diffusible. At equilibrium, the concentration of carboxy methyl cellulose, $[R^-]$ is 1.2×10^{-3} gram equivalent/liter and that of salicylate ion $[D^-]$ is 6.0×10^{-3} on one side. Compute the ratio of salicylate ion on the two sides of the membrane sac at equilibrium.***

$$\frac{[D^-]_o}{[D^-]_i} = \sqrt{1 + \frac{[R^-]_i}{[D^-]_i}}$$

$$= \sqrt{1 + \frac{12 \times 10^{-3}}{6 \times 10^{-3}}}$$

The ratio of the drug = 1.73

4. ***In the normal body, the concentration of plasma protein is 16 mEq/liter and that of the chloride ion is 113 mEq/liter. What is the ratio of chloride ions across the interstitial membrane (i.e., $fluid_{(outside)} \rightleftharpoons plasma_{(inside)}$)?***

The ratio of chloride ions is given by

$$\frac{[Cl^-]_o}{[Cl^-]_i} = \sqrt{1 + \frac{[R^-]_i}{[Cl^-]_i}}$$

Substituting the values

$$= \sqrt{1 + \frac{16}{113}}$$

= 1.07 to 1

5. ***Compute the ratio of concentration, at equilibrium, of diffusible benzyl penicillin ions (drug ions) outside to those of inside a semi-permeable membrane sac, when the concentration of a non-diffusible anionic polyelectrolyte inside the sac is 12.5 × 10^{-3} g.Eq /liter and that of benzyl penicillin outside the sac is 3.20 × 10^{-3} mole/liter.***

$$\frac{[D^-]_o}{[D^-]_i} = \sqrt{1 + \frac{12.5 \times 10^{-3}}{3.20 \times 10^{-3}}}$$

= 2.22 to 1

2. **Rheology**

6. ***It requires 40 seconds for a certain volume of water of density 1g/cm^3 to flow through a capillary viscometer and 614 seconds for an equal volume of a glycerin solution having a density of 1.12 g/cm^3. What is the viscosity of this glycerin solution at 25°C? The viscosity of water at 25°C is 0.01 poise or 1.0 centipoise.***

Time (t) for water to flow = 40 sec

Time (t) for glycerin solution to flow = 614 sec

Density of glycerin = 1.12 g/cm^3

Density of water = 1 g/cm^3

The relative viscosity of glycerin solution is,

$$\frac{n_i}{n_w} = \frac{\rho_l\, t_l}{\rho_w t_w}$$

$$\frac{n_l}{n_w} = \frac{1.12 \times 614}{1 \times 40}$$

= 0.172 poise

7. ***The time for water to flow through an Oswald pipette at 20 °C was 297.3 sec. the density of water at this temperature is 0.9982 and the density of a sample of olive oil is 0.910 g/ml. the viscosity of water at 20 °C is 1.002cp and the viscosity of the sample of olive oil is 84.0 cp. How long will it take for the oil to flow through the Oswald pipette at 20 °C?***

Time of flow for water

$$t_w = 297.3 \text{ sec}$$

Density water $\rho_{w=0.9982\ g/ml}$

Density of oil $\rho_{o=0.910\ g/ml}$

Viscosity of water $\eta_{w\ =1.002\ cp}$

Viscosity of oil $\eta_{o=84.0\ cp}$

Time of flow for oil

$$= \frac{\eta_o}{\eta_w} = \frac{\rho_o\, t_o}{\rho_w t_w}$$

$$\frac{84}{1.002} = \frac{0.910 \times t_o}{0.9982 \times 297.3}$$

$$= t_o = \frac{84}{1.002} \times \frac{0.9982 \times 297.3}{0.910}$$

$$= \frac{24928.25}{0.912} = 27333.6$$

or 7.59 hours

8. ***The torque produced by a Newtonian oil at 30 °C, when studied in cone-plate viscometer using large cone was found to be 120 at an rpm of 55. The instrument constant c is reported to be 1.168. Compute the viscosity of the oil.***

$$\eta = c.\frac{\tau}{v}$$

Substituting the values,

$$\eta = \frac{1.168 \times 120}{55}$$

$$= 2.55 \text{ poise}$$

9. ***Acetone was found to have a viscosity 0.313 centipoise at 25°C when determined using Oswald viscometer. It's density at 25°C is 0.988 g/cm³. What is the kinematic viscosity? What is the relative viscosity of acetone with respect to water whose viscosity is 0.8904 centipoise (cp) at 25°C ?***

Kinematic viscosity of acetone

$$= \frac{Viscosity}{Density} = \frac{0.313}{0.788}$$

$$= 0.397 \text{ centi pose} / (\text{g/cm}^3) \text{ or}$$

0.397 centistokes

Relative viscosity of acetone is $= \frac{\text{Viscosity of acetone}}{\text{Viscosity of water}}$

$$= \frac{0.313}{0.8904} = 0.352\ (dimensionless)$$

10. ***An o/w mineral oil emulsion was found to show plastic viscosity when analyzed in the cone-plate viscometer. Calculate the plastic viscosity of the emulsion using the data; torque, T = 110 at an rpm of 200 and T_f = 25 at rpm of zero, and c = 1.168. Also calculate the yield value f for the emulsion,***

Plastic viscosity, U

$$= C.\frac{T - T_6}{v}$$

Substituting the values,

$$U = \frac{1.168\ (110 - 25)}{200}$$

$$= 0.50 \text{ poise}$$

The yield value is given by

$0.122 \times T_f$, if large cone is employed in the cone and plate viscometer.

$$= 0.122 \times 25$$

$$= 3.1 \text{ dynes/cm}^3$$

11. A concentrated suspension consisting flocculated particles was found to have an yield value 5000 dynes/cm.^{2} At shearing stresses (F) above the yield value f the shearing stress was found to increase linearly with G, the rate of shear. If the rate of shear is 150 per sec when F was 8000 dynes/cm.^{2} Calculate the U, the plastic viscosity of the suspension.

Plastic viscosity, $U = \frac{(F-f)}{G}$

Substituting the values into the equation,

$$U = \frac{8000 - 5000}{150}$$

$$= 20 \text{ poise}$$

12. A newly formulated ointment base was studied at 20°C in a cone-plate viscometer whose instrumental constant c is 6.277 cm^{-3}. At a cone velocity v of 125 rpm, the torque, T was 1287 dynes.cm. The torque T_f at the shearing stress axis was found to be 63.5 dynes.cm. Calculate the plastic viscosity and yield value, if C_f is 113.6 cm^{-3} for the medium size cone.

Plastic viscosity, $U = C\frac{T-T_f}{v}$

Substituting the values

$$U = 6.277 \times \frac{(1287 - 63.5)}{125}$$

$$= 61.44 \text{ poise}$$

Yield value (f) is

$$F = c_f \times T_f$$

$$= 113.6 \times 63.5$$

$$= 7214 \text{ dynes /cm}^2$$

13. The following data were collected when a sample of zinc oxide in liquid petrolatum was analyzed at 25°C in a Stormer viscometer. w = 1800 g, w_f =1420 g, v = 500 rpm, and K_v = 50. What is the plastic viscosity in poises of this sample?

Plastic viscosity, U, is

$$U = K_v \frac{(w - w_f)}{v}$$

Substituting the values

$$U = 50 \times \frac{(1800 - 1420)}{500}$$

$$= 38 \text{ poises}$$

3. Coarse dispersions

14. If 1 ml (or 1cm³) of mineral oil is dispersed into globules with a volume-surface diameter d_{vs} of 0.01µm (10^{-6} cm) in 1 ml or (1cm³) of water, what will be the surface area of the dispersed oil globules and what will be the work input or surface free energy change in breaking the oil into globules or droplets?

The surface area increase is given by the formula

$$S_v = \frac{6}{d_{vs}}$$

Substituting the values,

$$S_v = \frac{6}{0.01} \; or \; \frac{6}{10^{-6} cm^2}$$

$$= 6 \times 10^6 \text{ cm}^2 \text{ or } 600 \text{ meter}^2$$

The work input is

$$w = Y_{o/w} \times \Delta A$$

Substituting the values, the work input or surface free energy change is

$$w = 57 \times 6 \times 10^6 cm^2$$

$$= 342 \times 10^6 \text{ cm}^2$$

$$= 34.2 \times 10^7 \text{ ergs}$$

$$= 34 \text{ joules or } \frac{34}{4.184}\ calories$$

$$= 8 \text{ calories (since 1 cal} = 4.184 \text{ joules)}$$

15. A hypothetical suspension contains 10^3 spherical particles of diameter 10^{-3} cm. assuming that the interfacial tension between the solid and the liquid, (γ_{SL}) is 100 dynes/cm, compute the total surface free energy.

Surface free energy is

$$w = Y\Delta\, A$$

Substituting the values,

For one particle, $w = 100 \times \frac{22}{7} \times (0.001)^2$

For 1000 particle, $w = 100 \times \frac{22}{7} \times (0.001)^2 \times 1000$

$$= 0.314 \text{ ergs}$$

16. A coarse powder with a true density, ρ_s of 2.44 g/cm^3 and a mean diameter, d of 100µm was dispersed in a 2% carboxy methyl cellulose dispersion having a density, ρ_o of 1.010 g/cm^3. The viscosity of the medium at low shear rate was 27 poises. Using Stoke's law, calculate average velocity of sedimentation of the particles of the powder in cm/sec.

Stoke's law is

$$v = \frac{d^2(\rho_s - \rho_o)g}{18\eta}$$

Substituting the values in the equation

$$v = \frac{(100 \times 10^{-4})^2(2.44 - 1.010) \times 981}{18 \times 27}$$

$$= 0.00029$$

$$\text{or} \quad 2.9 \times 10^{-4} \text{ cm/sec}$$

Sedimentation rate of particles is 2.9×10^{-4} cm/sec

17. Using Stoke's law, compute the velocity of sedimentation in cm/sec of a sample of zinc oxide having an average diameter of 1μm and a true density ρ_s, of 2.5 g/cm³ in a suspending medium having a density, ρ_o of 1.1 g/cm³ and a Newtonian viscosity of 5 poise.

$$\text{Stoke's law, } v = \frac{d^2\,(\rho_s - \rho_o)g}{18\,\eta}$$

Substituting the values in the equation

$$v = \frac{(1 \times 10^{-4})^2 \times (2.5 - 1.1)981}{18 \times 5}$$

$$= 0.0000015 \text{ cm/sec}$$

$$\text{or } 1.5 \times 10^{-7} \text{ cm/sec}$$

18. The average particle diameter of calcium carbonate in aqueous suspension is 45μm. The densities of calcium carbonate and water respectively are 2.8 and 0.997 g/cm³. The viscosity of water is 0.009 poise at 25 °C. Compute the rate of fall, v for calcium carbonate samples of different porosities, ε of 0.95 and of 0.5. The n value is 19.73.

First, we have to find the average velocity (v) by using Stoke's law

$$v = \frac{d^2\,(\rho_s - \rho_o)g}{18\,\eta}$$

$$v = \frac{(45 \times 10^{-4})^2 \times (2.7 - 0.997)981}{(18 \times 0.009)}$$

$$= \frac{0.0338}{0.162}$$

$$= 0.21 \text{ cm/sec}$$

Modified equation for Stoke's law is

$$v' = v\, \epsilon^n$$

Taking logarithms on both sides of the equation,

$$ln\, v' = ln\, v + n\, ln\, \epsilon$$

For $\epsilon_1 = 0.95$

$$ln\, v' = ln\, 0.21 + 19.73\, (ln\, 0.95)$$

$$ln\, v' = -1.5606 + 19.73\, (-0.0153)$$

$$= -1.5606 - 1.012$$

$$ln\, v' = -2.5726$$

$$v' = 0.076 \text{ cm / sec}$$

For $\epsilon_2 = 0.5$

$$ln\, v' = ln\, 0.21 + 19.73\, (ln\, 0.5)$$

$$= -1.5606 + 19.73\, (-0.6931)$$

$$= -1.5606 - 13.67$$

$$= -15.2306$$

$$v' = 2.43 \text{ K } 10^{-7} \text{ cm / sec}$$

It should be noted that at low porosity (ϵ) values (i.e., for 0.5), the sedimentation is hindered leading to small v' value.

19. The concentration of sodium oleate (soap) at the surface of a mineral oil emulsion (o/w) was found to be 0.02 mole per liter of oil. The globules were found by a microscope method to have a mean diameter of 1.0 µm (1× 10^{-4} cm). Calculate the mean area of one soap (sodium oleate) molecule at the surface of an oil globule.

Number of sodium oleate molecule is

Mole × Avagadro's number

$$0.02 \times 6.02 \times 10^{23}$$

$$= 1.204 \times 10^{22}$$

Surface area of globule is

$$\pi d^2$$

$$= \frac{22}{7} \times (1 \times 10^{-4})^2\ cm$$

$$= 3.14 \times 10^{-8}\ \text{cm}$$

Area per molecule

$$= \frac{3.14 \times 10^{-8}}{1.20 \times 10^{22}}$$

$$= \frac{3.14 \times 10^{-30}}{1.20}$$

$$= 2.60 \times 10^{-30}\ \text{cm}^2$$

20. Consider an o/w emulsion containing mineral oil with a specific gravity of 0.90 dispersed in an aqueous phase having a specific gravity of 1.06. Let the particle have an average diameter of 5μm and the external phase has a viscosity of 0.5 poise and the gravity constant is 981cm/sec². What is the velocity of creaming in cm/day? If the particle size is reduced by 5 times i.e., from 5μ m to 1 μm, what will be the velocity of creaming per day?

Applying stoke's law

$$v = \frac{d^2\,(\rho_s - \rho_o)g}{18\,\eta}$$

$$= \frac{(5 \times 10^{-4})^2 \times (0.90 - 1.05) \times 981}{18.05}$$

$$V = -4.1 \times 10^{-6}\ \text{cm / sec}$$

The minus is – (4.1×10^{-6}) indicates upward creaming since the internal phase density is lower than the external phase.

Since 24 hours/day contains 86400 sec, the rate of creaming –v, if the globale size is 5 μm

$$-v = 4.1 \times 10^{-6} \times 86400\, sec/day$$

$$= 0.35\ cm\ /\ day$$

If the diameter is reduced from 5 mm to $1\mu\, m$,

$$v = \frac{(5 \times 10^{-4})^2 \times (0.90 - 1.05) \times 981}{18.05}$$

$$= -\frac{0.0000014715}{9}$$

$$= -\ 0.0000001635$$

$$= -\ 1.6 \times 10^{-7}\ \text{cm/sec}$$

$$-v = 1.6 \times 10^{-7} cm/sec \times 86400\ \text{sec/day}$$

$$= 0.014\ \text{cm/day}$$

The upward creaming is 0.35 cm/day if the globule size is 5 μm and for 1μm globule size, it is 0.014 cm/day.

21. Mineral oil was dispersed to form o/w emulsion containing globules constituting a total surface area of 10^8 cm^2. If the presence of an emulsifier results in an interfacial tension between oil and water is 5 erg/cm^2, what is the total surface free energy of the system in calories?

$$w = \text{area} \times \text{surface tension}$$

$$= 10^8\ \text{cm}^2 \times 5\ \text{erg/cm}^2$$

$$= 5 \times 10^8\ \text{ergs}$$

$$1 \times 10^7\ \text{erg is equal to 1 joule}$$

Therefore, is terms of joules

$$\frac{5\times10^8}{1\times10^7} = 5 \times 10$$

$$= 50\ joules$$

Since 1 calorie is 4.184 Joule, the total surface free energy of the system in calories is

$$\frac{50}{4.184} = 11.95 \; calories$$

$$or \; 12 \; calories$$

22. ***What is the amount of soap (sodium sterate) in grams for a 100 cm³ emulsion containing oil globules of 1 μm (or 1 × 10⁻⁴ cm) diameter. The amount of oil in the emulsion is 50 cm³. The molecular weight sodium sterate is 306.46 grams.***

    a) ***What is the surface area of each globule (the diameter is 1 μm)?***

    b) ***How many soap molecules can be placed on the surface of each oil globule or droplet to cover it with a layer of one molecule thick, if the cross-sectional area of a soap molecule is 25Å²?***

    c) ***How many oil globules are formed in the 100 cm³ emulsion?***

    d) ***How many soap molecules are required to cover all the globules with a monolayer of soap globules?***

    e) ***What is the weight in grams of each soap molecule?***

    f) ***How many grams of soap are required to cover all the globules (of 50 cm³ oil) with a monolayer of soap molecules?***

(a) Surface area of globule is given by

$$\pi \, d^2$$

Surface area of each globule of oil $= \frac{22}{7} \times (1\mu m)^2$

$$= 3.14 \; \mu m^2$$

In terms of centimeter

$$= 3.14 \times (10^{-4})^2$$

$$= 3.14 \times \; 10^{-8} \; cm^2$$

Surface area of each globule is $3.14 \times 10^{-8} \; cm^2$

(b) Cross sectional area of each molecule is 25 $(\text{Å})^2$ and in terms of centimeter 25×10^{-8} cm^2

Then, the number of soap molecules covering each globule of oil is

$$= \frac{Surface\ area\ of\ the\ globale}{Cross\ sectional\ area\ of\ each\ molecule}$$

$$= \frac{3.14 \times 10^{-8}}{25 \times (10^{-8})^2}$$

$$= \frac{3.14}{25} \times 10^{-8} \times 10^{16}$$

$$= \frac{3.14}{25} \times 10^{-8} \times 10^{16}$$

$$= 0.1256 \times 10^{8}$$

$$\text{or } 12.6 \times 10^{6} \text{ or } 1.26 \times 10^{7}$$

(c) Number of oil globules per 1 ml of oil is given by

$$N = \frac{6}{\pi \rho d^3}$$

$$= \frac{6}{3.14 \times 0.9 \times (10^{-4})^3}$$

$$= \frac{6}{2.826} \times 10^{12}$$

$$= 2.1 \times 10^{12} \text{ globules / ml}$$

Number of oil globules produced from 50 ml is

$$2.1 \times 10^{12} \times 50$$

$$= 1.05 \times 10^{12}$$

$$= 1.05 \times 10^{14} \text{ globules}$$

(d) Number of soap molecules to cover 1.05×10^{14} globules i.e. all the globules in the emulsion is

$$1.05 \times 10^{14} \times 1.26 \times 10^{7}$$

$$= 1.32 \times 10^{21} \text{ soap molecules}$$

(e) Weight of each soap molecule is

$$\frac{Molecular\ weight\ of\ sodium\ searate}{Avogadros\ number}$$

$$= \frac{306 \times 46}{6.02 \times 10^{23}}$$

$$50.9 \times 10^{-23} \text{ gram/molecule}$$

Or, approximately

$$50 \times 10^{-23} \text{ gram/molecule}$$

(f) Number of grams of soap molecule (i.e. sodium stearate molecule) to cover all the oil droplets in the emulsion is

$$50 \times 10^{-23} \times 1.32 \times 10^{21}$$

$$= 50 \times 1.32 \times 10^{-23+21}$$

$$= 50 \times 1.32 \times 10^{-2}$$

$$= 50 \times 1.32 \times 10^{-2}$$

$$= 66 \times 10^{-2}$$

$$= 0.66 \text{ gram of sodium sterate}$$

23. ***A series of mineral oil was prepared using various combinations of Span 80 and Tween 80. The Span-Tween ratio of the best formulation was found to be 40/60. Compute the HLB of this mixture (or combination). Span 80 has an HLB of 4.3 and Tween 80 an HLB of 15.0.***

    Fraction of Tween 80 present in the mixture is 0.6 and hence, the HLB contribution by Tween is $0.6 \times 15 = 9$

Fraction of span 80 present in the mixture is 0.4 and hence, the HLB contribution by span 80 is $0.4 \times 4.3 = 1.72$

HLB of the mixture is, then

$$1.72 + 9 = 10.72$$

24. Calculate the required HLB (RHLB) for oil phase in the following o/w lotion

Light Mineral oil	***- 10g (HLB =11)***
Petrolatum	***- 25g (HLB = 8)***
Stearic acid	***- 15g (HLB = 17)***
Bees wax	***- 5g (HLB = 10)***
Preservative	***- 0.2g***
Water	***- 42.8g***

In the above formula, mineral oil, petrolatum, stearic acid and Bees wax form the oil phase. The total amount is $10 + 25 + 15 + 5 = 55$ g

HLB contribution by mineral oil is,

$$= \frac{10}{55} \times 11 = 2$$

HLB contribution by petrolatum is $\frac{25}{55} \times 8 = 3.6$

HLB contribution by stearic acid is $\frac{15}{55} \times 17 = 4.6$

HLB contribution by Bees wax is $\frac{5}{55} \times 10 = 0.91$

RHLB for oil phase is $2 + 3.6 + 4.6 + 0.91 = 11.11$

25. Compute the CMC of a mixture of two surfactants A and B. the CMC of surfactant A is 8.1 $\times$ 10^{-5} mole/liter and that of B is 15 $\times$ 10^{-5} mole/liter. If mole fraction of A (x_1) is 0.75, what is the CMC of the mixture?

The mole fraction of A = 0.75

The mole fraction of B = 1-0.75 = 0.25

The formula used for the calculation is

$$\frac{1}{CMC} = \frac{X_1}{CMC_1} + \frac{X_2}{CMC_2}$$

$$\frac{1}{CMC} = \frac{0.75}{8.1 \times 10^{-5}} + \frac{0.25}{15 \times 10^{-5}}$$

$$CMC\ of\ the\ mixture\ is\ \frac{1}{10926}$$

$$= 9.5\ \times 10^{-5}\ mole/liter$$

26. *The fraction of the drug, indomethacin released from a gel formulation at 250 minutes is 0.50. Compute the diffusional coefficient n, if k = 3.155% /minute.*

Since the rate is represented in percent, the fraction release should also be expressed in percentage units and it is 0.50 × 100 = 50%

The fractional release `F', of a drug from gel at time `t' is given by

$$F = kt^n$$

Taking natural logarithms on both sides of the equation,

$$\ln F = \ln k + n \ln t$$

$$n = \frac{ln\ F\ - ln\ k}{ln\ t}$$

$$= \frac{ln\ 50 - ln\ 3.155}{ln\ 250}$$

$$= \frac{3.9120 - 1.1489}{5.5215}$$

$$= 0.5004 \ or \ 0.5$$

As the exponent n = 0.5, the equation becomes

$$F = kt^{1/2}$$

This indicates the drug release is a Fickian modal or Fickian diffusion.

Note: Fickian diffusion: The fractional release F of a drug from a gel at time t may be given by

$$F = \frac{M_t}{M_o} = Kt^n$$

Where M_t is the amount released at time t, M_o is the initial amount of drug, k is the rate constant and n is a constant called diffusional exponent. When n=0, t^n=1 and the release F is of zero order. If n = 0.5, Fick's law holds and the release is represented by square root of equation. Such a release is called Fickian diffusion. Values of n greater than 0.5 indicates anomalous diffusion (non-Fickian diffusion)

27. ***Assume the interfacial tension of a particle of drug in aqueous vehicle is 100 erg/cm², its molecular weight is 200 g and the temperature of solution is 30°C***

  a) ***Compute the supersaturation ratio c/c_o that is required for the crystals to grow. The radius (R) of the particle is 5μm (or 5×10^{-4} cm) and its density is 1.3 g/cm³.***

  b) ***Compute the supersaturation ratio, when the particle is covered by a polymer and the pore radius, R of the polymer at the crystal surface is 6×10^{-7} cm.***

(a) The super-saturation ratio C/C_o is given by Kelvin equation

$$ln\frac{C}{C_o} = \frac{2\,YM}{NKT\rho R}$$

Where K is Boltzmann constant and the Nk value is given by 8.314×10^7 erg/deg mole.

Substituting values in the equation,

$$ln\frac{C}{C_o} = \frac{2 \times 100 \times 200}{(8.314 \times 10^7) \times 1.3 \times (5 \times 10^{-4})}$$

$$= 0.0024$$

$$\frac{C}{C_o} = anti\ ln\ of\ 0.0024 = 1.002$$

(e) $ln\frac{C}{C_o} = \frac{2 \times 100 \times 200}{(8.314 \times 10^7) \times 1.3 \times 303 \times 6 \times 10^{-7}}$ when covered by polymer

$$= 2.036$$

$$\frac{C}{C_o} = \text{anti ln of } 2.036 = 7.66$$

Note: In the case of (a), there is slight oversaturation (i.e. super-saturation) at which crystal growth will occur.

In the case of (b), the super-saturation must be 7.6 times larger than the solubility of the drug for the crystalline particle to grow. In other words, the point at which super-saturation occurs is greatly increased due to the covering of the crystals by the polymer added.

The crystal growth occurs as a result of addition of small particles to the crystals. The polymer is believed to cover the crystal preventing the access of small particles to the crystal to grow. The degree of super-saturation depends on the pore left over by the covering of polymer on the crystal. Smaller the pore, greater is the super-saturation point.

4. Micromeritics

28. From number distribution data a sample of powder, it was found that d_g (the geometrical mean diameter) and σ_g (the geometrical mean deviation) were 5.012 and 1.66 respectively.

Using Hatch-Choate equations, find the statistical diameters d_{ln} and d_{vs} and the d'_g for the powder.

$d_g = 5.012$ µm; $\sigma_g = 1.66$ µm

$\log d_{ln} = \log d_g + 1.151\log^2 \sigma g$

$= \log 5.012 + 1.151(\log 1.66)^2$

$= 0.7000 + 1.151(0.2201)^2$

$= 0.7000 + 1.151(0.0484)$

$= 0.7000 + 0.0731$

$= 0.7731$

d_{ln} = antilog of 0.7731 = **5.93µm**

$\log d_{ln} = \log d_g' - 5.757 \log^2 \sigma g$

$0.7731 = \log d_g' - 5.575\ (0.2201)^2$

$\text{Log } d_g' = 0.7731 + 5.757\ (0.484)$

$= 0.7731 + 0.2786 = 1.051$

d_g' = antilog of 1.051 = **11.24 µm**

$\log d_{vs} = \log d_g + 5.757 \log^2 \sigma g$

$= \log 5.012 + 5.757\ (\log 1.66)^2$

$= 0.7000 + 5.757\ (0.2201)^2$

= **9.52 µm**

29. ***From weight distribution data of a sample of powder, it was found that d_g' and σ_g were 10.4 and 1.43 µm respectively. Using Hatch-Choate equations, find the statistical diameters d_{ln} and d_{vs} for the powder.***

$\log d_{ln} = \log d'_g - 5.757 \log^2 \sigma_g$

$\log d_{ln} = \log 10.4 - 5.757\ (\log 1.43)^2$

$= 1.0170 - 5.757\ (0.1553)^2$

$= 1.017 - 0.1388$

$= 0.8782$

d_{ln} = antilog of 0.8782 = 7.55

d_{ln} = **7.55 μm**

$\log d_{vs} = \log d'_g - 1.151 \log^2 \sigma g$

$\log d_{vs} = \log 10.4 - 1.151(\log 1.43)^2$

$= 1.017 - 1.151(0.1553)^2$

$= 1.017 - 0.0277$

$= 0.9823$

d_{vs} = antilog of 0.9823 = 9.6

= **9.6 μm**

30. What is the specific area S_w based on weight of the particles of a sulfathiazole powder having a particle density of 1.5 g/cm³ and the average diameter of 2μm? Assume the particles are perfect spheres.

$$S_w = \frac{6}{\rho d_{vs}}$$

Substituting the values

$$S_w = \frac{6}{1.5 \times (2 \times 10^{-4})\ cm}$$

$$= 2 \times 10^4\ cm^2/g \quad \text{or} \quad 2\ m^2/gram$$

31. What is the total surface area in 1 cm³ of 4 g of a local anesthetic powder in which the particles have an average diameter d_{vs} of 2 × 10⁻⁴ cm and a true density of 2 g/cm³. Assume the particles are perfect spheres.

$$S_v = \frac{6}{d_{vs}}$$

Substituting the values

$$= \frac{6}{2 \times 10^{-4}} = 3 \times 10^4$$

Total surfaces = S_v × Volume of particles

$$= 3 \times 10^4 \times \frac{4}{2} = 60000\ cm^2$$

$$= 6\ m^2$$

32. A sample of charcoal powder was analyzed in BET apparatus before and after activation and V_m (volume of nitrogen gas in cm^3) values obtained were 3.4 cm^3/g and 260 cm^3/g respectively. Calculate the specific surface of the charcoal before and after activation.

Before activation

$$S_w = \frac{A_m\ N}{M/\rho} = V_m$$

$For\ Nitrogen\ gas\ \frac{A_m N}{M/\rho} = 4.35\ m^2\ /\ cm^2$

Specific surface of charcoal before activation is

$$S_w = 4.35\ \times 3.4$$

$$= 14.8\ m^2/g$$

Specific surface of charcoal after activation is

$$S_w = 4.35\ \times 260$$

$$= 1131\ m^2/g$$

Note: In activation of charcoal by heating, the already adsorbed particles on the surface of particles are desorbed (i.e., removed) Hence, the surface area is increased from 14.8 to 1131 m^2/g for the adsorption of nitrogen molecules.

33. Calculate the porosity of a sample of aluminum oxide having a true density of 4.0 g/cm^3, when 75 g of this powder was placed in a graduate cylinder, the powder was found to have a bulk volume V_b of 62 cm^3

Total porosity of a refers to the voids between the particles.

Void space = bulk volume – true volume

$$= 62 - \frac{75}{4}$$

$$= 43.25$$

$$Porosity = \frac{Void\ space}{Bulk\ volume}$$

Porosity $(E_{total})\ in\ fraction = \frac{43.25}{62}$

$$= 0.6975 \text{ or } 0.70$$

Porosity is usually expressed in percentage

$$\text{i.e., } 0.70 \times 100 = 70\%$$

34. If the weight of a tablet is 0.2626 g and its bulk volume is 0.0836 cm^3, what is the bulk density?

Bulk density of the tablet $= \frac{Weight}{Bulk\ volume}$

Substituting the values $= \frac{0.2626}{0.0836} = 3.14$ g/ cm^3

35. Calculate the percent porosity of a sample of a powder that has a true density of 2.70 g/cm^3. When 324 g of this powder was placed in a graduate cylinder, the powder was found to have a bulk volume of 200 ml (cm^3).

Void space = Bulk volume – True volume

$$= 200 - \frac{324}{2.70}$$

$$= 80$$

Porosity (E_{total}) in percentage is

$$\frac{Void\ space}{Bulk\ volume} \times 100$$

$$= \frac{80}{200} \times 100 = 40\%$$

36. The true density of aspirin powder is 1.37 and the granule density is 1.33. What is the porosity or percent void space within the granule?

$$\text{Porosity } (\epsilon) = 1 - \frac{grasule\ density}{true\ density}$$

$$= 1 - \frac{1.33}{1.37} = 0.03$$

Expressing in percentage

$$0.03 \times 100 = 3\%$$

37. The true density of a powder mixture is 3.203. When compressed into tablet after granulation process, the granule density was found to be 3.138. What is the porosity of the tablet?

$$\text{Porosity } E_{intraparticle} \text{ of tablet } = 1 - \frac{grasule\ density}{true\ density}$$

(granule density is tablet density)

$$= 1 - \frac{3.138}{3.203} = 0.02$$

Expressing in percentage

$$0.02 \times 100 = 2\%$$

5. Kinetics

38. The first order rate constant for the decomposition of ampicillin at 35°C and pH 5.8 is 2×10^{-7} sec^{-1}. The solubility of ampicillin is 1.1 g/100 ml. If a suspension of the drug containing 2.5 g/ 100 ml is prepared,

a) Calculate the zero-order rate constant, k_o

b) Calculate the shelf life, i.e., The time required for the dug to decompose to 90% of its original composition at 35°C

c) If the drug is formulated as a solution instead of a suspension at the same temperature and pH, what will be its shelf life?

(a) $K_0 = K \times A_o$

Where K_o = zero order rate constant

K = first order rate constant

A_o = Amount of drug initially in solution

$$K_o = 2 \times 10^{-7} \times 1.1 \text{ g/100 ml}$$

$$= 2.2 \times 10^{-7}$$

(b) Shelf-life is the time to decompose to 90% or by 10%. When the concentration of suspension is 2.5 g (100 A_o) t_{90} is

$$t_{90} = \frac{0.10\,[A_o]}{K_o}$$

$$= \frac{0.10 \times 2.5}{2.2 \times 10^{-7}}$$

$$= 0.113636 \times 10^{7}$$

$$or\ 1.13 \text{ to } 36 \times 10^6 \text{ seconds}$$

$$or\ 13.2 \text{ days}$$

(c) Original concentration C_o (or A_o) of the drug, formulated as solution, is 2.5 g/100 ml.

The concentration remaining (c) at the end of shelf-life is $2.5 \times \frac{90}{100} = 2.25 \frac{g}{100} ml.$

The first order rate constant is 2×10^{-7} / sec. Then t_{90} is given by the equation.

$$t_{90} = \frac{2.303}{k} \log \frac{C_o}{C}$$

$$= \frac{2.303}{2\times10^{-7}} \log \frac{2.5}{2.25}$$

$$= 526700\ seconds$$

$$\text{Or} = 6.1 \text{ days}$$

39. The initial stage of decomposition for a new drug according to a consecutive reaction was found to be first order. The initial concentration (c_o) of the solution was 0.050 mole/liter and after 10 hours at 40℃, the concentration (c) was 0.015 mole/liter. Calculate the specific rate at 40℃ and what is the drug concentration after 2 hours?

Specific rate constant K is given by the formula

$$K = \frac{2.303}{t} log \frac{C_0}{C}$$

$$= \frac{2.303}{10} \times 0.5224$$

$$= 0.120\ hr^{-1}$$

The concentration after two hours i.e. when t = 2 hours

$$= log\ c = log\ C_o - \frac{Kt}{2.303}$$

$$log\ c = log\ 0.050 - \frac{0.120 \times 2}{2.303}$$

$$= -1.3010 - 0.1042$$

$$c = antilog\ of - 1.4052$$

$$= 0.039 \text{ mole liter}^{-1} \text{ sec}^{-1}$$

40. A new drug product is found to be ineffective after it has decomposed by 30%. The original concentration of its sample was 5.0 mg/ml. When assayed 20 months later, the concentration was found to be 4.2 mg/ml. Assuming that the decomposition is first order, what should be expiration time? What is the half-life of the product?

$$log\ c = log\ Co - \frac{Kt}{2.303}$$

$$K = \frac{2.303}{20}.\ \log\frac{5}{4.2}$$

$$= 0.11515 \times 0.0755$$

$$= 0.0087 \text{ or } 8.7 \times 10^{-3}$$

The concentration remaining after it has decomposed by 30% is 100 – 30=70%

% of drug remaining is

$$5 \times \frac{70}{100} = 3.5\frac{mg}{ml}$$

$C_o = 5$, $C = 3.5$, $K = 0.0087$, $t = ?$

$$t = \frac{2.303}{K} log \frac{5}{3.5}$$

$$= 264.7 \times 0.1553$$

$$= 41 \text{ months}$$

$t_{1/2}$ for first order reaction is

$$t_{1/2} = \frac{0.693}{K}$$

$$= \frac{0.693}{0.0087}$$

$$= 79.6\ months$$

41. In the saponification of ethyl acetate at 25 ℃, the molar concentration of sodium hydroxide remaining after 75 minutes was 0.00552. the initial concentration of ester and of base was each 0.01 M. Calculate the second order rate constant and the half-life of the reaction.

The second order rate constant, K when equimolar concentrations of two reactants are involved, is given by

$$K = \frac{1}{at}\left(\frac{x}{a-x}\right)$$

$$a = 0.01; x = 0.00448; t = 75\ minutes$$

$$a - x = 0.01 - 0.0048 = 0.00552$$

$$K = \frac{1}{0.01 \times 75} \times \frac{0.0048}{0.00552}$$

= 1.082 liter mole/min

$$t_{\frac{1}{2}} = \frac{1}{ak} = \frac{1}{0.01 \times 1.082}$$

= 92.4 minutes

Table for conversion of Percentage into Probit Values

%	0	1	2	3	4	5	6	7	8	9
0	-	2.67	2.95	3.12	3.25	3.36	3.45	3.52	3.59	3.36
10	3.72	3.77	3.82	3.87	3.92	3.96	4.01	4.05	4.08	4.12
20	4.16	4.19	4.23	4.26	4.29	4.33	4.36	4.39	4.42	4.45
30	4.48	4.50	4.53	4.56	4.59	4.61	4.64	4.67	4.69	4.47
40	4.75	4.77	4.80	4.82	4.85	4.87	4.90	4.92	4.95	4.97
50	5.00	5.03	5.05	5.08	5.10	5.13	5.15	5.18	5.20	5.23
60	5.25	5.28	5.31	5.33	5.36	5.39	5.41	5.44	5.47	5.50
70	5.52	5.55	5.58	5.61	5.64	5.67	5.71	5.74	5.77	5.81
80	5.84	5.88	5.92	5.95	5.99	6.04	6.08	6.13	6.18	6.23
90	6.28	6.34	6.41	6.48	6.55	6.64	6.75	6.88	7.05	7.33

www.ingramcontent.com/pod-product-compliance
Lightning Source LLC
LaVergne TN
LVHW082019150826
845671LV00005B/210

9789395039383